BILL FRANK'S

forever young

HARPERRESOURCE

AN IMPRINT OF

HARPERCOLLINS*PUBLISHERS*

BILL FRANK'S

forever young

100 AGE-ERASING TECHNIQUES

BILL FRANK

This book is intended to be informational and by no means should be considered a substitute for advice from a medical professional, whom the reader should consult before beginning any diet or exercise regimen and before taking any dietary supplements or other medications. The author and publisher expressly disclaim responsibility for any adverse effects from the use or application of the information contained in this book.

"The Guy in the Glass" on page 218 is by Dale Wimbrow.

BILL FRANK'S FOREVER YOUNG. Copyright © 2003 by Bill Frank. All rights reserved. Printed in the United States of America. No part of this book may be used or reproduced in any manner whatsoever without written permission except in the case of brief quotations embodied in critical articles and reviews. For information address HarperCollins Publishers Inc., 10 East 53rd Street, New York, NY 10022.

HarperCollins books may be purchased for educational, business, or sales promotional use. For information please write: Special Markets Department, HarperCollins Publishers Inc., 10 East 53rd Street, New York, NY 10022.

First Edition

Designed by Ellen Cipriano

Printed on acid-free paper

LIBRARY OF CONGRESS CATALOGING-IN-PUBLICATION DATA

Frank, Bill, 1943–
    Bill Frank's forever young : 100 age-erasing techniques / Bill Frank.
        p.   cm.
    Includes index.
    ISBN 0-06-019837-0 (alk. paper)
    1. Longevity. 2. Aging—Prevention. 3. Rejuvenation. I. Title: Forever young. II. Title.
    RA776.75.F735   2003
    612.6'7—dc21
                                                        2002024149

03 04 05 06 07 WB/RRD 10 9 8 7 6 5 4 3 2 1

*This book is dedicated to all of us,
considered to be ordinary people, who share
dreams of extraordinary accomplishments and who
have the faith to believe these dreams can be fulfilled.
We are what we think we are and what we believe is
what we will achieve.
If you believe you can do it, you will do it.*

contents

acknowledgments

This book was written by a very ordinary man for the vast majority of us everyday people who want to understand how we can extend not just the length of our lives, but how we can improve the quality of the lifetime we are given. And we also want this information explained in terms we can easily understand and put into practice.

I could not have completed this task without the support and assistance of some very extraordinary people who have so generously contributed their time and wisdom to me over many years. It is these individuals who are the true authors of the material I have reported in this book. Their contributions to my life have made me what I am today. It is they who have taught me so much about remaining Forever Young.

TO THE PHYSICIANS

I must begin with Dr. Ernie Vandeweghe. This very special man could be listed in several categories for his contributions to my life's work. His wisdom about life alone gives him elite status. He captured one of life's great lessons in this quote: "I believe it's important in life to know what you don't know." Think about the wisdom in that statement for a moment. Ernie once said that the three R's we are taught in school should stand for respect, responsibility, and recreation. He said teaching those three R's to children would give them all they require to be successful. You need look no further than his family to know that he practices what he preaches. His wife Colleen is a former Miss America contestant. His son Kiki is a former All-American basketball player from UCLA, and after several years as a high-level performer in the NBA is the current GM of the Denver Nuggets. His son Bruk is a world-class performer on the beach volleyball circuit. His daughter Tauna was a three-time Olympian in swimming and volleyball. And his daughter Heather has followed in her father's footsteps as a very successful M.D. Thank you, Ernie.

To L. Cass Terry, M.D., Ph.D., Pharm.D., professor of Neurology, Medical College of Wisconsin. You'll meet Cass in my book. He is responsible for the chapter on the brain. He is a very special man who has taught me so much about the human body and the miracles that can be done with it. My greatest joy is that he numbers me among his many friends. It is an honor I don't take lightly. Thank you, Cass.

To Dr. David Leonardi, medical director of Cenegenics Medical Institute in Las Vegas. For his major contribution not only with the chapter in this book on hormone therapy, but for helping me to understand safe and practical ways of slowing the aging process.

To Dr. Alan Mintz, founder of Cenegenics Medical Institute, for making it possible for thousands of people around the world to slow the aging process. His commitment is second to none in his field. I also wish to thank John Adams and the entire staff at Cenegenics who put service and excellence above financial considerations.

To Dr. Marc Saginor of Los Angeles, Dr. Jim Shortt of West Columbia, South Carolina, Dr. William Malarky of The Ohio State University Medical Center, Dr. David Zipfel of Cincinnati, Ohio, and Dr. Arnold Segredo for their contribution to my overall knowledge.

To Dr. Nick Huston, Dr. Bill Joseph, Dr. Richard Menke, Dr. Larry

Hutta, and Dr. Wes Rosenthal for being there with total support when it was most needed.

TO THE ATHLETES

And I must preface this by saying that I cannot possibly list them all, and for that I apologize in advance. The ones I have to mention are the ones who were so much more than just training partners or casual acquaintances. There was Brian Downing of the California Angels. He is like a brother to me. His friendship, support, and belief in what we were doing and his willingness to speak out in favor of it (he is a very shy man) are things I will never forget. God bless you, Brian.

To Lance Parrish, the Detroit Tiger great. What makes Lance so special is not only his performance on the field but the quality of his character off the field. Lance's commitment to his wife and family always comes first. Lance never let a friend down and has a true and pure spirit. A man of similar character is Nolan Ryan. Nolan showed me that a man can be a great athlete, husband, father, and all-around great human being regardless of star status. Nolan never looked down on anyone, but offered a helping hand to many. And my thanks also to Rod Carew, legendary hitter, who showed me how to deal with injustice and adversity with dignity. He always knew who he was and what he wanted to accomplish.

And to all the other hundred or more professional baseball players who helped me understand their unique set of challenges in life and the many ways of dealing with them, I give my thanks. I taught them to lift weights, but I received so much more in return.

To basketball greats Bill Walton and Kiki Vandeweghe for demonstrating the positive results of playing for a great coach like John Wooden. I would acknowledge more athletes if space here were unlimited. You know who you are and I thank you.

TO MY BUSINESS ASSOCIATES

To Dan Levin, entertainment attorney and talent management. Dan should also be listed in the friends category. However, without his business acumen my television show *Bill Frank's Forever Young* would not have been on the Fox Health Network for two years. There would also not have been a book contract, so I guess he belongs here in business associates. But Dan, you mean so much more to me than just being my attorney. Believe it or not, it *is* possible for an attorney to remain a good and decent human being!

To Jerry Sellman, my personal business attorney for 14 years and my friend for life. He is a fine human being and will always have a place in my heart.

To David Halley, who has mothered over me in business the past six years, handling all the things time would not permit me to do. David, you did them well and with love and loyalty.

To Dan Adami, for your faith and friendship. To Pat Henry, for faith when only faith would do. Share the success, Pat! To Jean Berry, a lady in every positive way that can describe a lady. She has devoted her life to helping others when the roads she was traveling were untested. She pioneered the marketing of Live Cell Technology in this country. I love her dearly and hope the Lord will give her the rewards she so richly deserves.

To Mike and Lisa Doseck, a truly faith-filled couple, for their unending support and belief in what we have tried to accomplish together and for being there in the trying times when events and people seemed to conspire against us.

To Bill Reishtein—I could write pages about this man and never do him justice. He has meant so much to my life during the past five years. He has become my right arm. Bill is an advertising executive of the highest caliber. He is truly a genius when it comes to understanding the marketplace. No man ever got inside my head or understood my thoughts as rapidly as Bill. He spent countless hours with me as I spoke into a tape recorder about events in my life that led to the writing of this book. Bill is directly responsible for talking me into this undertaking. It is he who took my original thoughts and largely composed the original introduction to the book. He also structured and wrote the outline of the book proposal to HarperCollins. He edited the chapter that was originally submitted for book approval. So if this book changes lives, part of that credit must go to Bill. The only thing Bill didn't do was live the life I have written about. Bill, I hope this book and working so closely with me on it, will lead you to practicing all the principles you learned firsthand while working with me. But Bill means so much more to me than his part in creating this book. He was the total right-hand assistant in the development of the Forever Young program. He, along with my daughter Kelly helped produce many of our TV shows. He also helped create my infomercials for the Bio-Back. So you see what I mean when I say I could write pages about him. Without him I would have had to hire four other people and still wouldn't have gotten the quality I get with him. What you will read in this book is the story of my life and all the wonderful people who have contributed to teaching me the principles of fighting off aging. Bill Reishtein had nothing to do with that knowledge, but without him, you would never have had the opportunity to read this material, which we all hope you will put into practice in your efforts to remain Forever Young. Thank you, Bill. You truly are my right-hand man.

TO MY FRIENDS

This one's easy—just reread every name up above and I will add a few here and you have the list. The problem is that here again I am bound to miss many who should be mentioned. I will try to cover those directly related to the field of health and wellness that I hold so dear to my heart.

To Jack LaLanne—do I need to say more? No, but I will. Is there a more inspirational man in the world when it comes to exercise and health than this great man? He is an icon, the guru of all gurus. We all have a defining moment in our lives somewhere. Some, like me, are lucky enough to have several along the way. A couple of years ago in Boston, the health-club owners of America were giving Jack a very special award and he was to speak to the crowd. I was asked to introduce Jack to the club owners and guests. I was thrilled, honored, and very humbled to be able to introduce this great man to the crowd. Before I could leave the stage during the standing ovation Jack was getting, he stopped me. We were taping this for my TV show and nothing was rehearsed. When the crowd silenced, Jack said the kindest words ever spoken of me. He told the crowd that I was the next fitness guru in America and that if there were more Bill Franks in the world it would be a better place to live. As the tears streamed down my face, I also heard Jack say, "But Bill, don't get too excited. I'm a long way from retiring!" The crowd roared, and I said a quick prayer asking God to give him at least another 25 years. Stick around Jack, you have motivated me for over 40 years, and millions of people owe a debt of gratitude to you— the king of fitness. We love you, Jack, and we need you. I thank you for your tireless commitment to the health of multiple generations of Americans. Long live the king!

To Tom Rucker for keeping me loose. To Brad "Bubba" Sorenson for always being a loyal supporter. To Michael and Wilma Cox for bringing a special form of love into my life. Your contributions to your fellow man will live long past your trip to eternity. You are special people who have created special products to benefit all mankind. Michael, you have invented so many things. The Bio-Back is not only your latest, but also your greatest. May God keep you in his loving arms.

AND TO MY FAMILY

Each in his own special way has contributed to this book. They have all made me very proud of them. They gave my life a meaning and a purpose. Some were great college athletes—even All-Americans—and some were scholars. All of them are now successful adults, each in their own way. My daughters have both been news producers for some of the largest networks in America. I have a son who taught himself all he needed to know about computers and is on the ground floor of one of the fastest rising companies in that industry. Another son is a musician, currently working on his second CD as a singer-songwriter. And my youngest son, only two years out of college, is doing super with one of the world's largest bank and mortgage companies.

I know it seems as if I am bragging, but I am not. During all of their lives they allowed me to be involved with their youthful activities when my time permitted. They helped keep me young. The real reason I told you the great things about them is so I could tell you about my best friend—and theirs—their mother and my partner for over 30 years—the ultimate parent. She raised them 24 hours a day, 7 days a week. When I was on the road traveling, she was mother, father, friend, and companion. Whatever these children are or whatever they may become, they owe it to her. Throughout the years, while keeping a perfectly organized household, she also found time to raise enormous sums of money for the causes of the Jr. Women's Clubs of America. As the local president of that organization, she was named woman of the year. This was just another example to her children that you can accomplish several things at one time if you put each in its place and give it proper time and attention. Over the years she also found time to write and edit the newsletters for my companies. They were always first-class and award-winning material. She has been extremely instrumental in the writing of this book. She has typed chapters for me, organized the materials for each chapter, and tried to make sure I was grammatically correct! The lady's name is Priscilla. Her nickname is Prissy. But I will tell you there has never been anything prissy about the way she goes about her tasks in life. Everything she has ever done has been done with passion and total commitment. I have learned much from my best friend and she has helped shape the belief system you read about in this book. I hope all of you have your very own special Priscilla in your life. Thank you, honey, for the best years of my life.

Bill Frank

BILL FRANK'S

forever young

introduction

Can the unrelenting rush of sand through the hourglass be reversed? Can the detrimental toll that time takes on your body be halted in its tracks and headed in the opposite direction?

Yes! Absolutely. Positively. We live in a marvelous time when science and proven techniques that require nothing more than a body of knowledge and a reserve of willpower have joined forces to create age-management programs that are next to miraculous.

If you're one of the 80 million baby boomers who are aging in life together, your whole approach to this life stage is probably the polar opposite of your parents. Old ideas about "aging gracefully," easing into retirement, pulling back from activity, heading for the rocking chair and the Geritol bottle have happily been put to rest. Baby boomers now expect to remain active, involved, productive, and energized into their 70s, 80s and beyond. This book gives you the resources to make certain you maintain the health, youthfulness, and vigor to support the kind of life you want to create.

I've spent my adult life pursuing the secrets to defying age. I've studied with the world's leading antiaging physicians and scientists. I've shared knowledge with the World Anti-Aging Council and leading developers of cutting-edge nutraceuticals. I've helped professional athletes such as Nolan Ryan, Ozzie Smith, Lance Parrish, Brian Downing, and numerous other professional baseball, basketball, and football players add years of peak performance to their careers. And I've taught thousands of average people, from all walks of life, how to turn back the clock.

My television show, *Bill Frank's Forever Young,* teaches viewers how they can take years off the way they look and feel. This book goes one step further. I've taken all of the knowledge and techniques I've discovered and put them into a comprehensive age-management encyclopedia—a definitive tour guide through the world of renewed youthfulness.

Underlying every idea in this book is my unwavering belief that we ought to experience each day and each year of life with vigor and vitality—live to the fullest all the way to our last day on this planet.

For nearly a half century, I've been learning and integrating into my life the age erasers detailed in this book. The result? Beyond a tremendous psychological and spiritual sense of well-being, I've been able to actually turn back my physiological age.

In Chapter One you'll see a portion of an actual letter from antiaging specialist, Dr. David Leonardi, of the Cenegenics Medical Institute in Las Vegas, Nevada, who, after thoroughly examining me, declared that my biological age is "literally two to three decades lower than my chronological age." Am I bragging? No, I certainly am not. What I am doing is letting you know how grateful and thankful I am that everything you will read in this book has been taught to me over numerous years by many generous people. The only thing I can pat myself on the back for is being smart enough to listen and learn from the brilliant people who have contributed to the content of this book.

The purpose of this book is to show you how to achieve similar age-reversing results.

In which aspect of your life do you want to erase the negative influences of age? Whether it is your appearance, your sex life, your athletic life, or your overall health, this book provides you with the information and tools you need. There is not one silver bullet. Rather, there is a menu of techniques and technologies from which to choose.

Hormone replacement therapy, life cell therapy, vitamin therapy, minerals and herbal supplements, homeopathic remedies, weight training, aerobic exercises, tai chi, yoga, prescription drugs, laser surgery—all of these can be part of an effective age-management effort. This book helps you carefully weigh each age-erasing technique, giving you the pros and cons—detailing the kind of results you can expect.

Maintaining youthfulness is a lifelong pursuit. But getting started is the most critical step of all. I know from experience the rush and exuberance you will feel from making the commitment to a Forever Young lifestyle.

I also know that, once you've started, the wonderful reaction you'll receive from those around you will provide the motivation to maintain your positive, youth-restoring lifestyle changes for the rest of your life. You'll get used to, "Mary, you're looking terrific, what did you do?" Or "C'mon, you're much too young to have an 18-year-old daughter." I'm confident that these uplifting and affirming responses will motivate you to try even more of the age erasers I've outlined for you.

There's a younger, more energetic, healthier you that's ready to emerge. I promise you that I will help bring it out, if you promise me you'll use this book to build a personalized age-management program that fits your lifestyle and goals.

Together, we can remain Forever Young. Turn to Chapter One, and let's get started!

one

forever young:
a way of life

Any 25-year-old would be exceptionally proud of the results of Bill's blood tests. Bill's cholesterol and lipid profile put him in the very lowest category of risk for coronary artery disease. Bill's hormone levels are at the pinnacle of the optimal range for a healthy male between the ages of 25 and 35. The same holds true for his bone density, lean muscle mass, and thickness of skin. Bill's biological age is literally two to three decades lower than his chronological age.

Dr. David Leonardi
Cenegenics Medical Institute
Las Vegas, Nevada

The preceding was written about me by Dr. David Leonardi, an antiaging specialist, after he had performed one of the most complete physical examinations I've ever experienced. So—what am I, some kind of genetic freak whose body just doesn't age in the same way as the rest of the human race?

I can assure you that I am not. I am no different than you, except that long ago I made the conscious decision to unlink my physiological age from my chronological age.

Over the years, I've used my body as a laboratory and testing ground for many of the age-management techniques I'm going to tell you about in this book. And I know literally hundreds of people who have gone through the same physiological "reverse aging" process that I have experienced.

I've taught these techniques to hundreds of professional athletes and celebrities, who work in arenas where the stakes for youthfulness and maximum performance are very high. I've helped them prolong their careers and extend their maximum earning years. Many of them have become close friends and we now enjoy staying young together.

The professional athletes I've trained and advised call me "Vigor Man." Not just because of my personality and approach to life, but because of the energy and vigor that I've helped them discover, or in some cases, rediscover. Just today, I spent two hours helping one of Hollywood's most successful action heroes, who is well past his 40th birthday, get ready for his next physically demanding film. My goal is for this book to provide you with exactly the same advice, techniques, and encouragement.

You may or may not be familiar with my previously mentioned television show, *Bill Frank's Forever Young.* I mention it again because the show is all about taking my audience on a tour of the amazing world of age-management ideas and techniques, and it has served as a firsthand testing ground for many of the things that I want to share with you in this book.

I've visited the famous Cenegenics Medical Institute in Las Vegas, where they are practicing leading-edge hormone replacement therapy. I've visited the Steadman-Hawkins Sports Medicine Clinic in Vail, Colorado, where they have rehabilitated and returned to active competition elite athletes such as John Elway, Dan Marino, Bruce Smith, Terrell Davis, Greg Norman, Picabo Street, and Monica Seles.

I've learned kickboxing, power yoga, tai chi, had oxygen facials, hot rock massages, and exfoliation treatments. I've shared bodybuilding and workout techniques with Mr. America and aerobics champions.

Along the way I've taken on some adrenaline pumping adventures, which as I was approaching 60 years of age *were lifetime firsts for me.*

They included skydiving, scuba diving, mountain biking, snowshoeing, downhill and cross-country skiing, and in-line skating. The last adventure led to surgery to reattach ligaments in my elbow that were torn during a spectacular fall . . . and I arranged for the surgery to be filmed too! I've also taped shows on laser eye surgery, hair replacement surgery, and various cosmetic surgeries, as well as covering one of the newest anti-aging techniques available today—live cell therapy. My point here, however, is don't be afraid to try something new. The willingness to explore and at least try new things in your life is all part of the Forever Young experience. Don't be afraid to try something different. I promise it will invigorate you!

All of these experiences and more—all of the ideas, all of the advice, and all of the medical advancements I've explored are covered in the various chapters of this book. I have attempted to cover them in depth, yet in an uncomplicated, mystique-busting form. This is not a textbook or a scientific journal. It is meant to be an easy-to-understand instruction manual for turning back your biological clock. The central focus is on action—action you must take now!

I believe in the power and potential of people to be their best. I believe that life is a gift and that not living to our full potential is an unforgivable squandering of a precious gift. I realize that it is not easy to take control of your life, your health, and your age. But I also realize, from firsthand experience, that when you do take control the rewards are remarkable!

You must make the conscious decision to separate the physical and the chronological in your life. Once you make that decision, your life and your health will embark on a new and wonderful course.

We have to start with a plan of action—a mapped-out course for us to follow. I've designated a series of "age erasers," a spectrum of proven successful techniques, to serve as directional signposts along your road to age management. I will serve as your coach, trainer, cheerleader, and guide as you follow my map to successful age management—the Forever Young way of life.

DECIDE TO UNLINK CHRONOLOGICAL AND PHYSIOLOGICAL AGING

In order to create a road map to age management and remaining Forever Young, we must first define the concept. What do we mean by For-

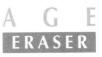

ever Young? Are we going to live forever? Are we going to live into eternity? Are we going to be like Methuselah? Is it a race to find out how many years we can actually stay alive?

Forever Young begins at the core of the mind. If you want to slow the aging process, you have to adopt your own counter-process. There is no one pill, no one therapy, and no one single approach that will accomplish your goals. Age management is an accumulation of changes and techniques—a lifestyle that you must design to suit you and your behavioral needs.

Look inward to your own likes and dislikes. You will find the things in your life that are part of your nature and things that go against it. Take an internal inventory and then choose from the menu of interventions that I am offering you. Create a way of living that is congruent with your attitudes and beliefs. Let's agree that you can make lifestyle changes that will affect you positively for the next 20, 30, 40, or 50 years!

The first thing you must do is develop an attitude that says, "I want to maximize my life." Just letting your health wander aimlessly from day to day and year to year won't cut it! You cannot just wait around and hope you stay fairly healthy from one year to the next, because left to chance you will ultimately "hit the wall." There are a plethora of health problems that will creep up on you and diminish your ability to enjoy life.

Instead, you must take control. Many people are perfectly comfortable managing an office, managing a sports team, managing their home—but are lost when it comes to managing their age. They feel that they must accept aging. In their minds, aging is a "natural" thing. They believe that those who fight aging are doing something very unnatural. This is absolute lunacy!

You maintain your home so that it will stand for many years. You take care of your car so that it will keep on running. You take care of your lawn, protecting it from predators and killers. You take care of these "things" in your life because you are trying to extend their life span and ensure that you get your money's worth from them. Yet so many people think that they should just accept the "natural" course of aging!

Yes, you will get older. Even I won't argue with that. But the inexorable deterioration that we call aging is not *natural* at all! And we have to stop accepting it as an inevitable part of life. You must develop a genuine desire to remain young.

In business, you have to be focused and have a passion for what you do. The most successful men and women on the planet have a road map in their minds of where they want to go and what they want to accomplish. They have the ability to see themselves in a successful business or at the top of their company. They see it completed and focus in on it. They plan ahead but are also not afraid to make changes along the way. They search out the most effective and efficient way to accomplish their goal.

There are older people who are admired because, even though they may have a hunched-over body, skin barely hanging on their frame, and no muscle tone at all, they still manage to project a great attitude toward life. They play cards, reminisce, visit friends, and seem to enjoy their lives.

But just imagine for a moment that if along with that great attitude, they had decided to take steps to assure that their circulation was still strong and healthy. They would be able to do more that just sit and talk about past life and loves; they would still be able to *make* love. They would be able to do this in their 80s and 90s. They would be able to take part in all of the activities they enjoyed in their younger days until their bodies just finally decided to shut down.

We don't know yet what the outer limits of the human life span can be. Scientists are telling us that if we can maintain ourselves for another 25 or 30 years, they will be able to give us another 50 years because of what they are learning about regenerating cells inside of the body. Scientists can do what they will, and they may be able to help you in the long run, but you will be far better off if you *take responsibility for yourself today.*

I believe that the human body is one of the greatest miracles ever conceived, and it is up to you to take care of that miracle, in the best way you know how, until the moment it is time to give it up for eternity. It all starts in your mind. You must develop an attitude of empowerment about what you want to do with your life and *your* body.

You must seek ways to slow the aging process and ways to erase some of the things that have already taken their toll. You must develop a value system that says: "I want to be able to enjoy my children and my children's children as a grandparent. I want to be an empty nester who still has enough energy and vigor to go dancing, take trips, and be productive so that I can make enough money to enjoy the years to come. I want to be super active in my 80s and 90s. I don't want to simply exist; I want to live with energy, enthusiasm, and passion."

You must develop a genuine belief that you are going to live each and every day of your life until it's time to go home. You must not simply be occupying space here on this earth. If you believe that your demise is already planned out for you, your diseases are predetermined, and no matter what anyone tries to teach you, this is your destiny—then this book is not for you. On the other hand, if you believe that you are going to live a long, full, and abundant life, and you simply need a tour guide to show you the pathways to optimum health and where to find all of the wonderful options available to prolong youthfulness, then keep reading.

I will help you to identify the biomarkers of aging and erase them from your life. I'll teach you how to eliminate the things that internally and externally are aging you at an unnatural rate. I will show you exactly how you can take control of your aging, turn it around, and start it running backwards. For those of you who are young enough and smart enough to begin this learning process at an early age, I will be able to help you slow the aging process down to a crawl. So let's get started!

UTILIZE A BREADTH OF FOREVER YOUNG INTERVENTIONS

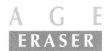

The road begins in the next chapter with the basics—getting your body ready for an infusion of youthfulness by getting rid of most negative influences. If this high-performance race car we call the body is dirty, clogged, and all gummed up, the eight-cylinder power plant may be running on only six or four cylinders. You must keep a clean machine, one that works well from the inside out.

So the first thing we'll talk about is how to detox your body. Most of us have put so many things in our body over the years that we have accumulated toxins and residue that cling to our internal organs. There are free radicals that accumulate on our cells forming "crust and rust" that keep our cells from performing properly, and that begin to harm our internal organs. It's easy to see how this process can contribute to the aging of our bodies. I'll tell you how to stop it.

The next thing we'll discuss is how to maintain your newly cleaned body. In Chapters Three and Four I'll tell you how to take 10 years of fat off of your body and tell you how to restore your youthful physique. This all begins with an understanding of how to take care of the inner workings of the body: keep it clean, keep it hydrated, and make sure that it gets plenty of fresh oxygen.

We are mostly made up of water. So we have to take a strong look at the hydration of all of our muscle tissue, our organs, and our cells. This is how you make sure that your body has the ability to perform at capacity. You want your body to take in a great deal of oxygen and efficiently use this oxygen to move blood to all of the organs so that they are getting the nutrients that they require. This is the channel of communication. This is the transportation center that circulates good health throughout your body.

You must be able to maintain your body in a state of homeostasis—a state that keeps your body in a perfect balance. All nature is about balance—harmonious balance. The goal is to keep your body hydrated, oxygen levels high, blood flowing, arteries and capillaries open, and circulation flowing.

You'll see the results in your mirror as you follow my advice in Chapter Five about how to save your skin. I take great pride in the look of my skin, especially my face. I don't think you will find a man in America whose skin, after 60 weather-beaten years, can outshine or outglow mine. I say this not to boast, but to let you know that I *do* have some secrets, and I'm going to let you in on them. I'm not a big proponent of cosmetic facial surgery, but for those of you who want to look into it, we'll cover some of the options available—from minor approaches to more severe and invasive ones.

You will want to make sure that you are continually active in your new Forever Young lifestyle. What you don't use, you lose—believe it! Exercise is essential to keep muscles, bones, and joints young. Our muscle and bone structures are precisely designed and mounted to function and work perfectly with each other. It's important to understand how to make the muscles strong and limber so they can function longer. It's just as important to understand how to take care of the skeletal structure, so that bones stay strong and straight and don't become brittle and break. Maintaining strong, healthy bones for life is our topic of discussion in Chapter Six.

Do you know the number-one function people are afraid of losing in their old age? The answer is memory. With the help of Dr. L. Cass Terry, the head of the Department of Neurology at a leading midwestern school of medicine, in Chapter Seven I'm going to take you through the subject of *nootropics*—the medical field that specializes in the study of new ways to improve mental acuity as we age.

You must constantly feed your brain. You must feed it with new information and stay on top of everything going on around you. What is important to you? Whatever it is, you have to feed it by reading about it. Challenge your mind. Keep it active. Do not let your mind become stagnant and decay from lack of stimulation. We need to understand the internal system that's fueling the body. What nutrients do we need? What keeps the body strong and supple? What feeds the heart and the lungs and organs of the body that contribute to prolonged health?

Do you feed your body only things that taste good and look great? Are they the nutrients that your body craves? Do you go fanatical one way or another? You must allow yourself a balance in life. You don't have to starve yourself or never enjoy anything that you want, but the key is moderation and making sure that your body gets the proper nutrients—the right fuel in the right balance.

After we've discussed the basic components in a proactive, Forever Young lifestyle, we're going to take your search for youthfulness much further in Chapters Eight and Nine. We're going to cover the antiaging properties of various vitamins, minerals, herbs, and antioxidants. We'll cover exercises that can give you back the figure or physique you enjoyed 20 years ago—and how you can cycle these exercises to make them dramatically more effective. We'll cover the kinds of foods that you should put in your body, and a very specific program to lose fat fast. We'll discuss sleep patterns and how important sleep is to youthfulness. We'll learn why I believe that the real fluid in the Fountain of Youth is adrenaline, and we'll discuss ways you can jump-start yours.

And with a restoration of your overall energy and vitality you can realize a change that will add years of happiness to your life by discovering a "recharged" libido and enhanced sexual performance, which we'll talk about in Chapter Ten.

Once you have made the commitment to integrate these age-management principles into your life, we'll be ready to explore some of the groundbreaking interventions that medical science is now making available to us.

Perhaps the most significant of these groundbreaking interventions is *hormone replacement therapy*—HRT—which many scientists believe is the key to reversing an array of the physiological symptoms of the disease we call aging. We lose these hormones at a rapid pace after the age of 25. A 60-year-old man or woman's body releases 67 percent fewer growth hormones than it did when they were in their 20s. HRT has been shown to reduce wrinkles, build bone mass, eliminate fat, improve cardiovascular health, increase energy, and improve sexual vigor. I've asked a leading antiaging physician, Dr. David Leonardi, to help us explore the potential benefits and possible risks of this therapy in Chapter Eleven.

In Chapter Twelve we are going to take a long look at the newest dimension of antiaging medicine called *life cell replacement therapy*. This cutting-edge technique is reported to rejuvenate and regenerate cell tissue in your body, giving you incredible new levels of youthfulness. Its proponents claim that the body's cells, tissue, and organs can return to levels enjoyed in your 20s and 30s. But is it for you? We'll take you through the pros and cons.

A major part of slowing down the aging process is finding your point of happiness in life. "Follow your bliss," as the saying goes. What is it that makes you happy? What drives you? Are you a goal setter? Are you a dreamer? Find out where dreams and goals fit in your life. If there is no balance between your dreams, your goals, and your reality, then being obsessed with them is a very quick way to age. And that's because this puts you under stress, and stress is one of the leading age promoters on the planet. Just ask any inhabitant of 1600 Pennsylvania Avenue. We routinely watch every president age a decade or more during each four-year term.

So seek out the right relationships in your life. Whatever or whoever it is that makes you happy, be sure they are a daily part of your life. This is very basic, but not very common. We'll discuss this further in Chapter Thirteen.

You must prioritize and determine which interactions in your life create a positive stimulus, so you can reap the benefits of a positive response in your body every single day. It's important to know where the combination of your mind, your body, and your spirit fits into your life. Although each one of the topics in this book has its own separate place and operates autonomously, they must all harmoniously interact in order to bring you total life and to undo aging.

Eastern civilizations have followed this mind-body connection for centuries. More and more physicians in the United States are working to heal disease with positive emotional and spiritual approaches to controlling the brain's neurotransmissions to the body. I believe that we should capture the magnificent power of the brain to constantly send our bodies signals of health, happiness, and youthful vitality.

A G E
ERASER

KNOW THE TRUE MEANING OF FOREVER YOUNG

You must *think* young in mind, you must *be* young in body, and you must *feel* a guiding and youthful spirit at all times to remain Forever Young. This book is about how you can unlock the natural secrets in your body. If you will have faith and try some of the things that you will read about, you will discover how you can put quality of life into each and every year that you live.

Whatever the "forever clock" is for you, I want you to live each and every one of those days. I don't want you to hit 60, and suddenly stop living, while science keeps you *existing* into your 90s. You might as well be locked up in a home because there is no real life for you.

If you are going to remain inside your body and on this planet until you are 105 years old, then for 105 years I want you to be able to get up out of your bed and play tennis, jog, travel, play with your great-grandkids, have fun, and if you want to have a physical relationship with your partner . . . just keep on loving until it is time for you to go.

This is the true meaning of Forever Young. *Not living forever, but forever living.*

two detox your body

W e're about to embark on a wonderful journey though the world of renewed youthfulness. I'm going to introduce you to groundbreaking vitamins and minerals, cutting-edge hormonal treatments, and age-retarding cellular therapies. You will learn about exercise routines that will give you back your physique, nutrients that will restore the healthy radiance of youth to your skin, and incredible herbs and nutraceuticals that will invigorate your sex life.

But before we go any further, I want you to stop and give yourself a metabolic clean slate. I want a clean canvas on which to paint a picture of a beautiful, new, more youthful you.

You probably don't want to think about all of the toxins, poisons, and physiological by-products that are clogging and choking your system. Artificial flavorings and colorings, environmental toxins, harsh preservatives and chemicals that permeate your water, air, and food end up lining your intestines and settling in your liver. They have become an unwanted component in your entire internal system of cells and organs.

When you are born, your body is pure and clean. Unfortunately, you spend the rest of your life filling it with foreign substances that slow it down, make it sick, and age it prematurely. Your body's purifying system, while wonderful and miraculous, just isn't equipped to keep up with this all-out toxic bombardment that is a result of living in today's biotechnical world.

You wouldn't dream of going decades without changing the oil in your car or the filter in your furnace. Yet you may not think twice about allowing a lifetime of toxins to set up shop in your cells and remain there forever.

Now is the time to detoxify and purify your system, and get your body ready for an infusion of health and energy. Detoxing your body is like cleaning out a messy closet or garage. It seems to get a lot messier before it gets clean. That's my way of letting you know that it could get a bit "gnarly" as your body rids itself of all of these toxins and impurities. But this lasts only a short time and then your body will be cleansed and in a much healthier physiological state.

I'm going to tell you about an array of methods to detox your body as the first component in your program to remain Forever Young. But before you begin your return to youthfulness, you should start by determining precisely what your current state of health is and what, exactly, is your body's physiological age.

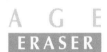

BEFORE CLEANING, GET A SCREENING

Before you begin any program—cleansing or otherwise—you need to know the current status of your body. I recommend a complete blood workup and health screening. Go get the testing done. Get your body screened. Find out your cholesterol levels, your lipid levels, and your hormone levels. You should also determine your bone density index, your body fat index, and your cardiovascular condition. You should know exactly what condition your body is in before you start any new program.

The saying in business is "You can't manage what you can't measure." The same is true for your health. Your health screen will tell you things about your health that you need to manage. It will give you a sense of your physiological age. For example, if your cholesterol level is higher than your testosterone level, I can safely say that's not the way you want to be aging. So you can work to turn it around.

How are you going to measure your progress if you do not understand your starting point? Everyone should have these blood tests done at least once a year to be safe. But I believe in being proactive. So I recommend at least twice a year, because we intend to monitor the results and intervene where needed. Personally, I have blood screening done as often as eight weeks and certainly never more than sixteen weeks apart. For me, it is always at least four or five times each year. I want to keep track of exactly what's in my bloodstream. I want to know the moment that there is something there that doesn't belong. If there is a problem, it will show up in the blood work. That's the telltale sign.

This is how I keep my immune system strong and my disease risk low. I never have a day that I don't feel positive, because I know that I am clean and healthy from the inside out. That's where life is lived— from the inside out. So make testing a part of your program. Get your blood workups done and understand exactly where your body is, so you'll have a good jumping-off point. Have it checked again 16 weeks later. If you are following our Forever Young program of detoxification, vitamins, minerals, antioxidants, exercise, and an array of additional age-management interventions, I know that you are going to look better and feel better at the time of your second test. And you'll have a numerical documentation of your progress—always an encouraging factor.

Your frequent health screening and blood tests will provide empirical evidence that your metabolism is getting younger. It will also tell you exactly which areas require further concentration. By the way, it's also fun to share with your physician, and watch his amazement at the dramatic improvement of your health and age biomarkers.

Every executive in my company gets a health screening the day they start working, and begin their Forever Young health program. Then, they get screened according to the above-mentioned schedule. Soon, I will have the youngest and healthiest company in America—and we will have ongoing records of our health screenings to prove it! I want to be able to say the same thing about my television viewers and about you, the readers of my book. If you need the names and addresses of good health-screening resources in your area, see the reference section at the end of this book. Now, let's detox.

A DISTILLED WATER FAST

Twice a month, I cleanse my system with a distilled water fast. When you give your body a period of time without making it work to digest and absorb your food, it utilizes this break in activity in a very positive way. It acts like a self-cleaning oven and begins to rid itself of the toxins and contaminants it has been collecting.

As you fast, you will begin to purify your blood. Your kidneys will also undergo purification as you continue to flush them. You should be drinking a large amount of distilled water, from 12 to 16 glasses per day. Do not use tap water or spring water. They are full of dissolved solids, minerals, and other contaminants.

Our goal now is to avoid introducing any of these elements into your system, so distilled water—which is nothing but water—is the best choice. In addition, toxins, free radicals, and poisonous elements in your body will magnetically bind to the molecules in distilled water, which greatly enhances the detoxification process. The liver, because it no longer has a lot of metals to deal with, will naturally cycle and purify itself and eventually filter out even more substances that shouldn't be in your body.

These poisons may not endanger your life immediately, but over the years will cause degeneration in your cells, organs, and tissues. The distilled water, first of all, will cleanse the kidneys and begin to clean out the intestinal tract as it moves through your system. It will pull toxins, poisons, and free radical systems from the upper and lower tract of the intestines and colon. These toxins may be destroying the walls of your cells and literally aging your organs before their time.

Many, many years ago a close friend of mine, someone that I recognize as the ultimate guru of the antiaging program—Jack LaLanne—taught me his detox program, and this is the plan I use to this day.

In the beginning, I started with 12- and 24-hour fasts, as you should too. Then I went to 36 hours. I would stop eating at 5:00 on Sunday evening and not eat again until 5:00 on Monday evening. Then I went from 5:00 on Sunday until 8:00 on Tuesday mornings, and then before I knew it, I could fast from 5:00 on Sunday evening all the way to Saturday morning of the next week. I was finally able to put in 120 hours plus, and it was truly an amazing feeling to clear my head and clear my body. I had incredible mental stamina and energy. My blood pressure would come down. My pulse rate would be lowered way down to the high 50s, and I was so calm and so clear thinking.

I would always break my fast with stewed tomatoes and then I'd have a nice fresh salad with just a squeeze of lemon juice on it. Then I would gradually start my normal diet again to put the protein back and begin regenerating my body tissue.

I still try to do this program twice a month—I fast from Sunday evening at 5:00 all the way up to Thursday morning, so I am actually going in excess of 72 hours. I sometimes fast for 96 hours, but I certainly do not recommend this to anyone reading this book, without first having a consultation with a physician. Before you go on any fast, you should consult with your physician, especially if you have any preexisting medical conditions. Start with a shorter duration to see how your body responds—then gradually extend your fasts.

As you get into the second day of your detox effort, you will begin to notice some very positive changes—after you get past being very hungry, which you will after about 24 to 26 hours. Most people feel an increase in vitality and greater energy—not only physically, but mentally and emotionally too. There will be a calmness about you. Frequently, allergies will be diminished because there are not a lot of toxins in your body bolstering or attaching to these allergies, and certainly there will be a de-stressing of your digestive functions.

After 36 hours, you should notice an improvement in mental clarity and memory. If you are able to make it to the 72-hour period, your body is not only eliminating toxins that have entered your body recently, but it is now extracting from stored toxins and stored metals as it begins to break up fat deposits in your body. Sometimes you will get a little bit light-headed as you are passing these toxins through your body.

By hour 72, your increased mental sharpness will be very pronounced. The mucus is cleared up from around the brain and other memory centers. Hormone secretion improves. The immune system is strengthened. You begin to feel like a ninja—totally tuned in to everything around you.

You are probably thinking, "Well, wait a minute. Won't I feel zapped and listless because I don't have food for energy?" You may feel this way at first. But, remember that you are detoxing your body. You are cleansing it of the things that are attacking it on the inside—of free radicals that are preventing your cells from receiving neurotransmissions and functioning to their full potential. You are scraping the corrosion off the "battery terminals" in your body. It only makes sense that you will feel a greater flow of energy.

Your immune system is strengthened during detox. Your blood, kidneys, and liver are all purified. They are purified because they are not combating all of the other unwanted foreign elements inside your body that are irritating it. You have increased vitality, because your body doesn't have to spend so much energy fighting off all of these toxins and irritants.

There are those who fast on distilled water or juice for as long as 21 days. I am not advocating that you start fasting anything near that or even 7 to 14 days. You will serve yourself well to start with a 24-hour fast once a week for two or three weeks. This is easiest if you begin your 24 hours right after dinner one evening, because by the time you get up the next morning you're already halfway there or more! Then you can try 30 and 48 hours and so forth until you are able to reach 72 hours once or twice a month.

I believe you should make fasting a regular part of your lifestyle. It plays a key role in keeping your body younger on the inside, and sets the stage for all of the wonderful nutrition and positive things we're going to add to your life.

Now, I'm going to review some ways to maintain the detoxification process when you are not in a fasting period. It is essential to realize that after your fast is over, you need to load up on your vitamins and minerals. You should adhere to a complete supplementation regimen. This should include the complete B complex family of vitamins—not just B_1 and B_2, but also B_6, B_{12}, choline, inositol, and riboflavin.

You need to have your antioxidants—especially vitamin C and vitamin E—and your minerals—zinc, copper, selenium, manganese, molybdenum, and magnesium. All of these vitamins and minerals are critical to maintaining good health, as you rebuild your body following your distilled water fast. (See Chapter Eight, Antioxidants Against the Diseases of Aging, for a complete explanation of these nutrients.)

I also recommend milk thistle, NAC (N-acetyl-cysteine), charcoal, and lactobacillus acidophilus. These are nutrients that help to detoxify the small intestines and colon.

Breaking your fast the proper way is also extremely important. When you stop fasting, your stomach will be smaller, so be kind to it and don't overload it right away. Drink some juice and have some stewed tomatoes or apples as your first solid food. A few hours later have some raw or steamed vegetables. Consuming these first will continue the process of flushing out your body. Eat more often, but make your portions small. After a day you can work back into your regular diet and begin to include proteins. But remember—you've just cleaned your body—so eat smart!

FIBER, GARLIC, LEMON JUICE, ALOE VERA, AND MORE

When you are not fasting, there are certain foods and supplements that can help you keep your system cleansed. Fiber, of course, is like a scrub brush that keeps your colon clean and keeps food moving through your system quickly. There is agreement from nearly all medical and scientific sources that fiber reduces the risk of colon cancer, by sweeping it clean, and keeping the toxins from spending any great length of time against the walls of your intestines.

Fiber is just the beginning. There are numerous other substances that can create wonderful cleansing in your intestines:

- ➤ **Garlic supplements** kill the parasites and harmful bacteria inside the system. They cleanse the mucus congestion in the body.
- ➤ **Lemon juice** also has an enormous cleansing effect in the colon.
- ➤ **Aloe vera** helps to heal colitis, diverticulitis, hemorrhoids, and irritable bowel syndrome. This is not just something new; it has been on the market for many, many years. There are a lot of claims made about aloe vera that are not substantiated—everything from enhancing muscle density to improving sexual performance. I don't believe these claims, and I wish the companies making these claims would stop. But, nevertheless, aloe vera is a wonderful detoxifier and is excellent for intestinal health. It should be part of your program, if not daily, at least weekly.
- ➤ **Spirulina** detoxes the blood and the bowels of the system. It's like a broom that sweeps right through. Once things have been broken up, it has a tremendous ability to sweep the toxins right out of your body.
- ➤ **Pau d'arco,** which is a South American herb, combats chronic yeast and fungal infections. It is an herb that every woman should take. Men hear about yeast infections and think that it's just a woman's problem, but yeast infections are inside our systems everywhere, and men have them too. It is highly advisable

for everyone to take the herb pau d'arco regularly to help eliminate yeast and fungal infections.

YOU WANT ME TO PUT COFFEE WHERE . . . ?

Viewers of my show know that I will do almost anything to help keep my body in a more youthful state, to enhance my health, and to improve the quality of my life. In many cases, I am a proponent of what I call "aggressive antiaging interventions." If you look at the poor physical condition of many people in their 60s, 70s, and 80s, you know that the aging process can be quite aggressive, so I believe in responding with just as much intensity.

I'm going to tell you about a technique that always elicits jokes and winces from people, but I can tell you it is a wonderful age eraser and promoter of good health. It's up to you if you're ready to go the distance in this area of detoxification. A friend of mine and an associate in my company, calls it the "Starbutts" program—a little takeoff on Starbucks, the coffee that you can find at every airport and on almost every corner in America today. The procedure we jokingly call "Starbutts" is a coffee enema, which, in all seriousness, is an extremely beneficial way to stimulate, cleanse, and detoxify your system.

Over 50 years ago during World War II, a well-known surgeon, Dr. Max Gerson, discovered a detox program while performing surgery on many soldiers who were mortally wounded in combat. Before performing surgery on the soldiers coming straight from the battlefield with devastating abdominal wounds, he used an enema procedure to cleanse their systems. After running out of pure water before a critical operation, he found, by accident, that his results were greatly enhanced when he detoxified their systems using, not water, but coffee. Much to his amazement, postoperative soldiers who usually required a great deal of morphine for pain now required less, and seemed to heal more quickly. This inspired Dr. Gerson to do many years of research on just exactly what took place during these unusual battlefield surgery incidents.

Dr. Gerson's battlefield experiences with coffee enemas became one of the techniques used at the Gerson Anti-Cancer Clinic, where alternative therapies are used to heal cancer victims. Dr. Gerson's detoxification theories have shown remarkable results. I had the pleasure of filming an episode of *Forever Young* at one of the clinics, which are now managed by Dr. Gerson's daughter, Charlotte. At age 80, Charlotte is as energetic, vibrant, and vigorous as a woman half her age. I fell in love with her principles, her ideas, and the kind of person she is. I loved the clinic's commitment to fighting cancer and other diseases, and their willingness to try alternative treatments.

The incredible detox diet that they give all of their patients—which includes natural vitamins and herbs, phytochemicals, juices and vegetable blends, and the previously mentioned coffee approach, has shown a wonderful ability to rid people of poisons and toxins that previously suffocated their bodies. It has also shown remarkable healing results among cancer victims.

Why is this process so important to me? Because with all of the alcohol people drink, all of the sugars they consume, all of the empty carbohydrates and fats that block their livers, and the cholesterol problems they have, a healthy, functioning liver is vitally important to good health. You must keep your liver clean and operating at maximum levels. One way this can be done is through the detoxification process of coffee enemas, which pull toxins from the liver and in so doing helps create a healthier spleen.

The clinic's detoxification programs have resulted in many "miracle" cancer cures. But I'm wondering, why wait until you get cancer to detoxify your liver and to keep your system pure? It's common sense that if you can keep free radicals out of your body, if you can keep your cells clean and protect them, your body is going to be stronger and you are certainly going to remain healthy longer.

I certainly agree with Dr. Elson Hass, director of the Marin Clinic of Preventive Medicine and Health Education in San Rafael, California, who said:

> I believe that the process of detoxification, through special cleansing diets as well as juice and water fasting, is the missing link to rejuvenating the body and preventing such chronic diseases as cancer, cardiovascular problems, arthritis, diabetes, and obesity.

However, I also believe that Dr. Max Gerson was way ahead of his time in realizing that it was one thing to fast and break up all the toxins and chemical poisons in our body, but it was even more important to then eliminate them and not create further damage to our intestinal tract and colon.

Seventy years ago Paul C. Bragg was teaching us that fasting broke all of the many dangerous chemicals loose. But imagine the power these chemicals have for a short period of time as they attempt to pass through our system on the way to being eliminated from our body. What danger could fasting do to other organs like our liver, kidneys, spleen, and our bowels in the process of this internal war going on in our body?

For years, many physicians would not recommend fasting because they could not be sure their ailing patients were well enough to handle this rapid and active detoxification process. How long would it take to eliminate these killers from our "homeland" and how much damage will be done as they exit our body? It's like any war. How many innocent must die before the last battle is won? How many organs will be pitted and how many cells damaged while the enemy is being driven from our bodies?

Max Gerson knew that we had to protect our homeland—our vital lower intestinal tract and organs—while we won this war. He discovered that coffee had properties that bound itself to toxins and escorted them out of the body. Through research and patient care he found that the coffee enema cleansed and protected the lower intestinal tract. It acted as a magnet and pulled the toxins off the liver, kidney, spleen, and other vital organs. It then acted as a healing compound to smooth the scales and scar tissue on body organs and in the colon, thus greatly reducing the risk of cancerous cells forming.

If you have never tried a coffee enema it may sound strange. But just think about this: whenever you are scheduled for a medical procedure that involves your gastrointestinal tract—stomach, intestines, colon—the first thing you are told to do is cleanse the system by drinking fluids and giving yourself enemas. You have to literally clear the way for the efficacy of the particular treatment and for the accuracy of the test result.

The logic is the same here. Why not try to keep your system clean and toxic free most of the time? A coffee enema once or twice a week may go a long way toward accomplishing this. If you want to read more about the Gerson therapy, and coffee enemas in particular, please see the reference section at the end of this book, visit your nearest library, or go online and type *Gerson therapy* into your search engine, and you will find all the information you'll need to decide if this age eraser is for you. I believe that once you understand the history behind the therapy and read more in-depth information as to how it works, you will not find coffee enemas such a strange thing.

It certainly makes sense to me that all of us would want to utilize at least some of these therapies *before* our body becomes diseased. In many ways, that is the definition of age management. My recommendation: Don't be afraid to try something different if the ultimate result is the creation of a more youthful internal environment for your cells and organs.

CHELATION THERAPY

As we graduate up the ladder of detoxification intensity, there is another process called chelation therapy—and its effectiveness can be phenomenal. Chelation is a very powerful detoxifying process that reaches right into the lymph nodes, the bloodstream, and the neurotransmission centers of the body. It quickly and dramatically removes excess metals and toxins from all of these areas. This therapy may produce excellent and lasting success for some people, so I am going to give you a brief explanation of how it works.

Chelation therapy involves intravenous infusion of EDTA (ethylene-diamine-tetra-acetic acid) over three to four hours, which binds to toxic metals and minerals and pulls them out of tissue so they are easily excreted. In a regime of eight to ten treatments the effectiveness of this therapy should reach its optimum level of success.

The word *chelation* derives from the original Greek word *chela* meaning the claw of a scorpion or crab. Simply put, chelation therapy works as the infused substance grabs the undesirable material, binding them together and thus enabling their removal from the body. *Bind* is truly the key descriptive word in this process.

The human body could not survive without the constant process and benefits of chelation. Here are perhaps a couple of easier to understand examples of chelation: When you use a water softener, you are chelating minerals out of the water with the infusion of salt. When you use detergent in your dishwasher or your clothes washer, the detergent chelates with minerals in the "dirt" and allows them both to be washed away by water. When you digest food, your body uses ingested protein to chelate with minerals and then transports the minerals to their intended destination within the body. Literally thousands of body processes constantly use chelation mechanisms.

That's just a simple layman's explanation of a complicated chemical process. It is not my intent, or even a possibility in this book, to tell you everything about this therapy. I urge you to do your own investigation into this therapy as well as any new therapy you may consider. Refer to my reference section at the end of this book for other sources of chelation information.

A word of caution: Some physicians with questionable knowledge and/or motives are convincing patients to take chelation treatments for one year or more. They are promoting health abilities well beyond its proven function to detoxify the body.

In my opinion, which is shared by many physicians and scientists that I respect, the ultimate benefit of the detoxification effects of chelation therapy are realized after eight to ten treatments. However, you may want to repeat the treatments every six to eight months for a couple of years if you have been abusing your body for a long time. The negative aspects of what has happened within your body did not take place overnight, and by the very nature of preconditioned habits, the average person will return to many of the same negative behavioral patterns that have always been practiced. This, in addition to the incredible amount of toxins, bacteria, and metals, etc., in our atmosphere, leads me to believe that taking eight to ten treatments a couple of times a year for two or three years can not only completely detoxify the circulatory system, but can help us alter our negative behavior patterns into those compatible with a healthy lifestyle.

A friend of mine, Dr. Jim Shortt of Columbia, South Carolina, has been treating his patients with chelation therapy for many years. He tells me that the number-one benefit of chelation therapy is the prevention or elimination of lipid peroxidation—the process wherein fat is oxidized, solidified, and retained as stored fat in the lining of cells, organelles, and blood vessels. Chelation eliminates this by binding the metals that catalyze these reactions. All cell membranes contain lipids, which ultimately solidify and not only drain the body of energy, but cause it to function well below expected capacity, adding to the aging process. Chelation therapy will not only break up and destroy the oxidated, stored fat cells in the body, but will also aid in preventing floating or liquid fat from ever accumulating as stored solid fat.

But I reiterate to you that eight to ten treatments at any one time are enough. Any additional treatments are unnecessary as it relates to detox, and are not proven to contribute to other health benefits. Excessive numbers of treatments are an abuse of a wonderful technique.

Chelation therapy has a powerful place in your age-management program because it is one of the most effective eliminators of free radicals within the body, and the elimination of these free radicals not only improves your overall well being, but also drastically slows the aging process. But please understand the finite nature of the need for treatments and the limits of its benefits.

TOLERATE A FEW UNPLEASANT DAYS

Some of the short-lived normal responses to detox include fatigue and headaches during the first three days, transient sleep disturbances, insomnia or excessive sleepiness, increased body odor, itchy skin, irritability, increased gas, bad breath, and hunger. But before you say "no way" and turn to the next chapter, remember, all of these conditions are short-lived, and none persist once your detox program is complete.

Don't forget, there are a lot of chemicals and fatigue products in your body that have been there for months or years. As a result, when they start exiting your body, there will be a short-term price to pay. But I assure you, you'll feel great knowing that you've purged all of that nasty stuff from your body!

There will be hunger initially, not only because you have stopped eating, but also because there is the additional secretion of hydrochloric acid and other products in your body. As substances break loose, your body reacts as if there is food, and goes into a digestive state with nothing to digest. The sleep disturbances are a result of all the substances that have been dormant breaking up during the night. They are not so easily passed, and that's why you must drink a lot of water during any detox program. Your skin itches because many toxins are pulling away from your skin inside your body, or they are pouring through your skin as a result of excessive perspiration. You will probably feel more confidant about your personal hygiene if you take warm showers and use a very good deodorant or antibacterial soap during this time.

Remember, all of the unpleasant attributes that are showing up now are a result of toxins that have been walking around with you day and night for years. After three days, a lot of them will be gone forever. None of these effects will continue after you complete the detoxification process. You just need to be strong and do the right thing for your system, keeping in mind the wonderful long-term benefits to you and your new lifestyle.

REBUILD AND MAINTAIN
YOUR NEWLY CLEANSED BODY

Once your body is cleansed and detoxed, its time to rebuild and maintain your body. That's really what the rest of this book is about. Begin a program of antioxidants and all of the other essential vitamins, minerals, and high-energy herbs, so the free radicals don't come back and get a grip on you.

Gear up your exercise program. Transform your diet with more healthy protein and less fat, sugar, and salt. Look into hormone regulation and all of the other new techniques that are safely restoring youthfulness to so many people.

Most important, as you go through all of the remaining stages of your program to remain Forever Young, *keep coming back to the principles and practices outlined in this chapter*. Keep up your detox program with regular fasts. Continue to have your health screenings and blood tests so you can track your progress and direct your future efforts.

Above all, always remember that your health and your age are in your control. Have some fun managing the process yourself—you will be delighted by the results.

Now that you have a nice, clean, healthy body on the inside, let's work on getting back the lean, healthy appearance you had a decade or two ago. In the next two chapters I'll show you how to melt away the fat you've spent the years since college collecting, and how to build back the youthful physique or figure you thought was gone forever.

three
how to lose
10 years of body fat

Please read this chapter with the following in mind: It expresses my personal opinion, which has been developed over the years from my experiences working with hundreds of athletes and celebrities who were trying to reach a specific goal, for a specific purpose, in a designated period of time. However, I must warn you that not all diets are suitable for everyone.

Before you begin this, or any dietary change, you should consult with your physician and receive permission to participate in a change of diet and vigorous exercise. If, at any time, you experience discomfort or pain that you believe is caused by dietary factors, STOP, and immediately see your doctor. Depending on your state of health as you begin a dietary change, your body may be adversely affected by a sudden increase in the amount of protein in your diet. This is not the norm, but you may have particular medical problems that you aren't even aware of at the moment.

The instructions, experiences, and advice presented here are in no way intended as a substitute for medical counseling. I am not there with you in person to assess your physical condition, and am not qualified to assess your medical status. So please, go see your friendly doctor and then come back and let's get started losing 10 years of body fat!

Although this is an unusual diet, there is nothing drastic about it calorie-wise. It is *not* a low-calorie crash diet. This is my eating plan for life. It is the one that I've taught to all those I love.

Let me be blunt. Excess body fat ages a body faster than any other lifestyle factor, with the exception of cigarette smoking. It ruins your health, negatively affecting just about every aspect of your life. A recent study from the Harvard School of Public Health found that men with a 42-inch waist were nearly twice as likely to experience impotence than men with a 32-inch waist. How often do you hear men with 45 inches of girth around their waists bragging about their love lives? Most women understand that men with a lot of excess fat often have circulation problems that prevent them from being good lovers or enduring lovers. In the same way, a woman who has allowed a roll of excess fat to accumulate around her midsection is not a stimulating or attractive partner to most men. And this is but one example of how excess fat is destructive to healthy living.

Many people in their 30s and 40s believe that it is inevitable to gain fat around the middle of their bodies at this stage of life. Maybe that is why it is called "middle age" they bemoan. This middle-age spread used to be considered a measure of one's success; but that was over a hundred years ago—in the "olden days" as my children would say! It is not a measure of success today, except for the fast food and junk food purveyors who prosper from our eating habits. Over 64 percent of us, or 98 million people, are overweight. If the average overweight person is carrying 10 extra pounds, that's nearly a billion pounds of excess blubber being carried around! This is not a pretty mental picture, especially when you consider the heavy burden that all of this fat places on our country's overall health, not to mention the very personal burden it places on your heart and your cardiovascular system.

A health club that I recently visited had a big, yellow, irregularly shaped piece of foam rubber about the size of a loaf of bread displayed on their counter. When I inquired about it, they told me that it was a realistic model of a pound of body fat. It doesn't take any great imagination to realize how two or three of these things could choke the life out of your body.

Why does this happen to so many of us? It's an unfortunate double whammy that seems to accompany this stage of life. As lifestyles become more sedentary, the body's metabolism slows down. To make matters worse, body fat is metabolically inactive, so the greater percentage of fat we add to our frames, the fewer calories we burn—leading to more unused energy in the form of fat. It's a vicious cycle that leads to millions who are dangerously overweight or obese.

Excess fat is a significant factor in a broad range of chronic diseases normally associated with aging—including heart disease, diabetes, impotence, and hypertension. A declining percentage of lean muscle mass also contributes to a decline in our aerobic capacity and our ability to maintain an increased metabolic rate to continually burn fat. An elevated percentage of body fat will eventually contribute to the loss of bone density—another negative health factor that we seem to accept as a part of "aging."

LIVE BY THE NUMBERS

I'm going to throw some statistics at you, which I hope will stick. These frightening statistics from the National Research Council, the National Cancer Institute, and the American Heart Association, speak volumes about the intertwined relationship between health, disease, longevity, and fat.

➤ Poor diet, especially one high in calories from fat, is associated with 60 percent of cancers in women.

➤ Lung cancer is five times higher in adults whose diets are high in saturated fats.

➤ Adults who consume a diet of 38 percent fat have 10 times the recurring rate of skin cancer as those who eat a diet with 20 percent fat.

➤ The risk for developing adult-onset diabetes is three times greater among individuals who are overweight.

➤ The American Heart Association credits fat with being the primary contributor to heart disease, which claims nearly one million lives per year.

➤ Studies show that blood pressure in adults increases sharply with weight gain from fat tissue, and decreases sharply with the loss of weight from fat tissue.

A G E
ERASER

Now consider these numbers: The mean body weight of Americans has increased 7.9 pounds over the past 15 years. Are we building up our muscles and so increasing our weight by spending more time at the gym? Sorry, that's not the case. The average American now loses 6.6 pounds of lean muscle mass each decade after their mid-20s. When you hear your mushy coworker boast that he weighs the same now as he did in college, you can assume that his body composition has merely converted from muscle to fat and that his health profile has declined right along with the percentage of lean muscle mass in his body.

LEARN YOUR FAT-TO-MUSCLE RATIO

The body-fat norm for middle-aged men is 16–18 percent. For women it's 24–26 percent. For people committed to the principles of Forever Young, which are to optimize health, vigor, and youthfulness, I recommend that men should keep their body fat at 12–14 percent and women should be at 18–20 percent. Women have been created to bear children; therefore, they have been given a little extra cushion and fuel. In fact, if a woman goes under 9 percent body fat, she is dangerously close to being someone who is going to have future health problems including difficulty bearing children. So don't go too far the other way.

Although you may have read about professional bodybuilders with 4 or 5 percent body fat, these are numbers that are reached by these men and women only prior to their competitions during the year. This is a dangerously low body fat level even to the competitive bodybuilder and could be life-threatening to the average person. Although body fat is dangerous at a high level, remember that there is also danger at the other end of the spectrum.

Body fat seems to creep up on people unnoticed, unless they happen upon an old photo or they attempt to squeeze into a suit or dress that they haven't worn in many months. They wake up one day and they have two to five extra pounds around their waist and they say, "That's not too bad." And then, in another couple of years, five or ten more pounds appear and they say, "Well, uh, I guess, uh, that's not too bad." Then, before they know it, they have crept closer and closer to the obese category, and their health is seriously compromised. Finally, one day they say "Oh, my God, that isn't me . . . Is it? I've got to do something about this!" The question should be, how do you *prevent* it? First, I will discuss how to accomplish this. Then I will address those unfortunate souls who have found themselves "over the top." I'll teach you how to get out of this state permanently.

DRINK WATER TO LOSE FAT

In other chapters you will hear me talk about water in your diet and its positive influence on your skin and other aspects of good health. Drinking plenty of water, preferably distilled, is also a very good way to lose fat. Many people neglect to keep their body adequately hydrated. Without a hydrated body, lactic acid, free radicals, and fatigue by-products (pyruvic acid, hydrochloric acid, etc.) that can interrupt circulation begin to accumulate. A lot of tension from stress in our daily lives comes into the body and interferes with the good homeostatic process of proper metabolism and fat burning. This literally allows pockets of fat (unused energy) to accumulate and also allows the body to go into a catabolic state, using muscle for energy instead of body fat.

Distilled water has a magnetic resonance effect that attracts toxins and poisons and pulls them out of the body. Tap water, with all its metals and gases, only adds to the complications. The elimination process that should be automatic actually slows down dramatically, and sometimes comes to a screeching halt. Toxins that should pass through the body do not pass, and a nasty accumulation takes place.

Fat pockets begin to accumulate in the midsection of our bodies, on our hips, around our buttocks and upper thighs, eventually creeping into the intestines, and then dangerously close to the heart. As the fat begins to form around our rib cage it hinders our capacity for free-flow breathing. The fat then continuously creeps closer to the most valuable organ in our body—the heart. So drink a great deal of distilled water. If you are inactive, drink at least a half ounce for every pound of your body weight. And if you are super active, you need to take in an ounce of water for every pound of body weight. This is the most significant anti-aging secret of all time. It is also one of the simplest, easiest, and safest ways to lose overall body fat. And it's good for you in so many other ways too.

Remember that 10 glasses of water is a minimum. I prefer drinking at least double that or about a gallon per day. Your body will retain water if it senses the possibility of being deprived, so drinking a lot will eliminate water retention, which will give you some immediate visible reward for doing something so healthy. Drinking a lot of water can also help suppress your appetite. Again, whenever possible, make sure the water you are so diligently drinking is distilled. This should become a staple of your antiaging, antifat age-management plan.

THE 60-PERCENT SOLUTION

The next thing we need to consider is the various ways different foods in your diet are digested in the body. Understand the specific dynamic action of foods: how much heat and energy your body produces in order to digest, assimilate, and convert the foods you eat into enzymes and energy.

Your body temperature rises only 4 percent when you eat fat. It rises 6 percent when you eat carbohydrates and 30 percent when you eat protein. What does this mean to you? First and foremost, if you eat 1000 calories of fat, by the time the stomach digests this you are still stuck with 960 calories in your body. If you eat 1000 calories of carbohydrates, by the time you digest it you are stuck with 940 calories in your system. If you eat 1000 calories of protein, by the time you digest it, only 700 calories remain. Almost one third, or 300 calories, have already been burned in the process of simple digestion. This is the reason a high-protein diet is far more effective in weight reduction programs than just eliminating carbohydrates or fats. When mixed with water, the protein is more readily absorbed by muscle tissue, and not stored as fat, as are unused carbohydrates and fats.

I encourage you to make 60 percent of your diet protein, which will leave you in the range of 30 percent carbohydrates and 10 percent fats. This is a higher percentage of protein than many diets recommend, but far from the so-called power protein diets that hopefully are a passing fad. Now, before you run to your library to compare these percentages to your old diet books, remember this is an *antiaging* diet. I recommend being more aggressive with your protein ratio, because I believe that building muscle is such a crucial component in your age-management plan. *I want to create change in your body, not facilitate the status quo.*

Remember that all muscle tissue or cellular regeneration is created by nitrogen, and the only source of nitrogen that your body can make use of is in the conversion of protein to nitrogen. If you wish to count them for antiaging reasons, the ratio is 6.25:1. In other words, if you consume 50 grams of protein, you will end up with 8 grams of nitrogen. Your heart alone requires 8 grams of nitrogen per day for proper functioning.

Can you imagine those individuals trying to consume only 40–60 grams of protein per day? The heart takes it all, and then it's no wonder our muscle tissue ages, our liver, spleen, pancreas, and other internal organs age more rapidly and cause more diseases and interruptions in our healthy lifestyles—all long before the heart calls it quits and ends the game for good.

That is why I recommend a gram of protein for every pound of lean body tissue, which equals the total weight of your muscle mass, bone density, and internal organs minus the weight of your fat tissue. If you are a 180-pound man with 15 percent body fat, that means you have approximately 153 pounds of lean body mass, and should be consuming 153 grams of protein each day. It's the same principle for a 120-pound woman. Simply deduct your percentage of body fat from your weight and consume a gram of protein for every pound. This will assure you that your heart will not be the only survivor. Instead, it will be thriving as the leader of the army of your internal organs marching forward with vitality, vigor, and a great zest for life and for staying young.

Of course, I'm trusting that you are complying with the other important parts of your age-management program, part of which is your exercise program. When you combine a higher level of protein intake with a regular exercise routine, especially weight training, you will produce the maximum fat loss/muscle gain effect that you desire. This is a crucial pillar in your age-management regime.

People are designed to live over 100 years. According to many scientists, the heart could give us 150 years of normal use if there were not so many factors that we put in its way. If we could only learn to increase our heart's longevity through exercise and clean living, instead of decreasing it with fat, poor nutrition, and other damaging environmental factors, we could get a lot closer to reaching our age potential. If we could create a perfect environment without crash diets, alcohol, fat, sugar, chemicals, and toxins—if we could stop interrupting our life span with external factors—we could come much closer to our dreams of remaining forever young.

EAT HEALTHY FATS AND THE RIGHT CARBS

The body needs fat to function properly. It is not only a lubricant, but is necessary for the proper functioning of your heart, the maintenance of skin tissue, and healthy hair. Have you ever noticed how overweight

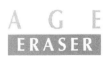

people often have glowing skin and a wonderful head of hair? These precious few positive qualities associated with being overweight come from the polyunsaturated fats, not the monounsaturated fats.

There *are* such things as healthy fats. They are the GLA fats, the omega 3s, and the omega 6s that the body and brain require. We talk more about this later when we discuss a healthy eating plan and some of the foods that are low glycemic, but at the same time provide you with enough fat and carbohydrates to sustain and balance your diet with protein.

Once you have accepted the fact that you should limit your fats to 10 percent, choose your carbohydrates very selectively. Do not eat empty carbohydrates. I am not a great fan of rice or bread or a lot of unnecessary sugary carbohydrates. I believe in consuming fresh fruits and vegetables. I recommend a program that allows you to have three to five servings a day—whether that be an apple or a banana or half a grapefruit. Some of these you can have at breakfast and the balance later. I limit my carbohydrates, but I have some of them in the evening. Carbohydrates in the evening often lead to a more restful night's sleep. However, do not consume insulin-elevating sugary carbohydrates, especially foods made with refined sugar like cookies and cake, which may leave you jittery and cause you to toss and turn all night long.

Protein is king in a diet that keeps you strong, healthy, and vigorous. It helps to increase your muscle density and works with your hormonal system. At the same time, it helps create body heat and elevates the metabolism, which aids in the burning of fat cells. A high-protein diet helps regenerate cellular tissue in the body, which requires nitrogen for maintenance. As I have previously stated, nitrogen only comes from protein, it does not come from fat or carbohydrates. With your protein consumption at 60 percent, you will find yourself on the leaner side, yet with a strong foundation upon which to build muscle.

Daily activity will help you keep fat off of your body, especially once you understand the amount of calories it takes to maintain your weight and the amount of caloric burn that is required to take a pound or two off. It requires 3000 calories worth of activity or a 3000-calorie deprivation to burn off one pound of fat. If you simply add 500 calories of activity over a six-day period, that's 3000 calories. So—if you just do an exercise that creates a 500-calorie burn over your normal daily activities each day, you could look forward to burning a pound of fat every week. If you've found yourself 10–15 pounds overweight, and you don't want to go to a gym and sweat it off, all you have to do six days a week is take a brisk one-hour walk at a fair pace. If your diet hasn't changed, you'll lose a pound a week. Is walking too slow or dull for you? The following will provide the same fat-burning result:

➤ A half-hour bike ride maintaining 20–25 miles per hour
➤ 35–40 minutes of rollerblading
➤ 45 minutes of fast-paced tennis
➤ *Walking* 18 holes of golf—no carts allowed!
➤ 35–40 minutes of weight lifting
➤ On a treadmill, a brisk walk of 45 minutes at 4 miles per hour will burn nearly 600 calories.

WORK YOUR ENTIRE BODY, NOT JUST YOUR MID-SECTION

If you want to lose fat and shed years, you must increase your physical activity level. If you don't want to do that, you should throw away this book! I realize my book is full of a variety of age-management techniques, but without this one, the rest are only fractionally valuable. So take a cue from the old Olivia Newton-John hit and "Let's get physical."

It's not good enough to take a 3500-calorie-per-day diet and reduce it to 3000 calories if you are only burning 2500 calories per day. Although your body requires a certain amount of calories in order to function, you must exceed that basic metabolic rate of caloric burn to lose fat.

There are various exercises for the entire body that you need to do, even if you are going to focus on fat around the middle. Remember that the best way to take fat off around the middle is not to specialize in abdominal exercises and leg raises alone. You must create an overall body caloric burn.

If you do an aerobic activity for 45 minutes, you will increase your sustained metabolic rate, which will continue from one to two hours after you have finished the activity.

If you spend an hour lifting weights and raise your metabolic rate, it will stay at that level for approximately three hours. The heart and the lungs will have to work and the neurological system will have to work. They will require energy. This energy will be provided by the continual caloric burning of fat, if you have been successful in keeping our calorie intake modest.

A G E
ERASER

Begin a complete body workout routine, in which you work yourself from the tips of your toes to the top of your trapezoid muscles in your neck and shoulders. Create an entire movement of fat depletion throughout the body. You want blood flow and circulation that stimulates the usage of fat as the energy source. You may do it with weights or aerobically.

A treadmill is an outstanding cardiovascular exercise, but it is not one of the great fat burners because most of the blood and most of the activity is taking place from the hips down. Some of the best aerobic training is done by cross-training or moving your arms and legs at the same time on a cross-country skiing–type machine or other cross-trainers. Cross-training requires activity in the upper back, the shoulders, the hips, the buttocks, and the waistline.

Once you have established that you are going to add an aerobic or weight-training program to create an overall caloric burn, you can then settle on specific abdominal exercises. This does not, however, include the old way, using sit-ups. Sit-ups not only can result in thickening your waistline, but also potentially create low back strain, or worse, damage to the tissue around your spine. Plus, if you are not adding aerobics or the caloric burn, you will only end up with a broader stomach with fat on the outside.

Beginning on page 35 you will find descriptions and demonstrations of my Forever Young Fat Burners. They include cross-training exercises, and a variation of abdominal exercises, leg raises, oblique work, and upper and lower back exercises. If you do 50 repetitions of abdominal work, then you should do a like number for the low back or lower spine. If you want a solid, strong midsection, then you must build a solid lower back to offset a great deal of this activity. Otherwise, you will experience low back pain and low back strain and you may find yourself in the doctor's office.

You must work the rectus abdominis area also. Check out the variations of leg lifts, side bends, and modest comfortable twisting routines I demonstrate for you. All of these are combined in the abdominal region for muscle toning that works in concert with the caloric burning of your aerobic exercises.

But remember, some cardiovascular exercises are better than others for fat burning. *Low intensity for long periods of time* will burn fat in the body most rapidly. Plus, as time goes by, this type of exercise is easier on your heart, your blood pressure, and your joints.

> ### CROSS-TRAINING AEROBICS

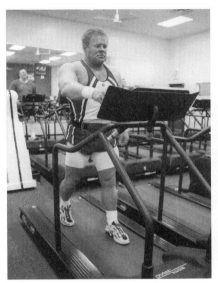

Treadmill: Use a combination of normal walking pace to a faster jogging pace.

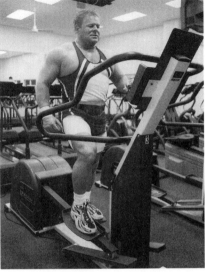

Stair Climber: Set resistance to work your heart 30–40 percent above your normal heart rate.

ABDOMINAL EXERCISES

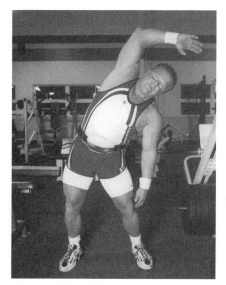
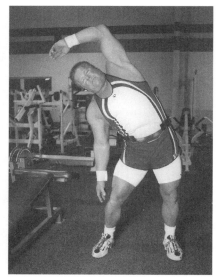

Side Bends for Oblique Area

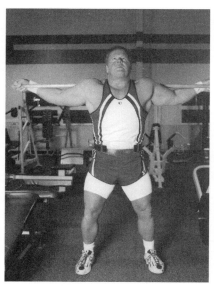
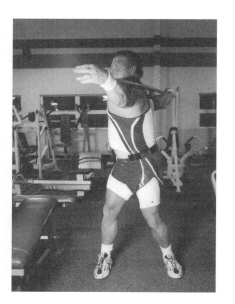

Twists for Overall Waist Reduction

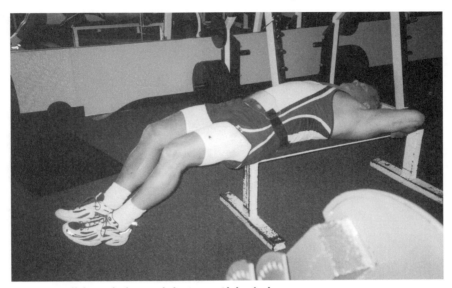

Leg Raises off the End of a Bench for Lower Abdominals

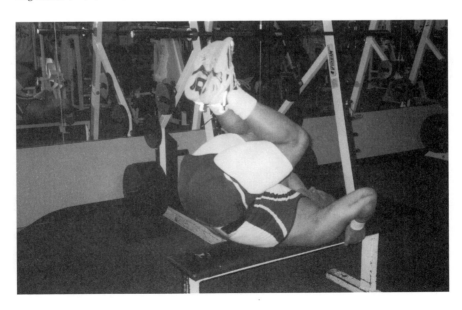

➤ **UPPER BACK EXERCISES**

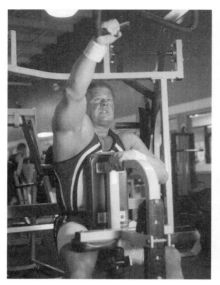
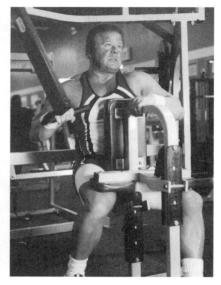

One-Arm High-Pulls (Do Both Arms!)

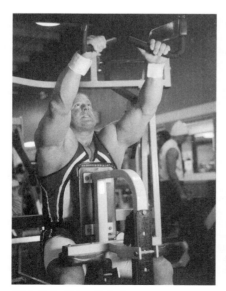
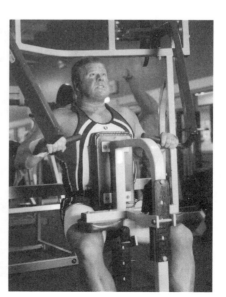

High-Pulls Using Both Arms

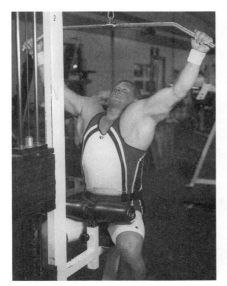
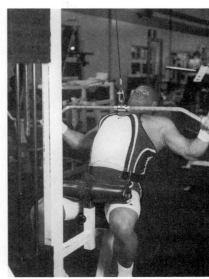

Front Lat Pull-Downs

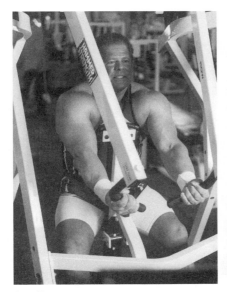
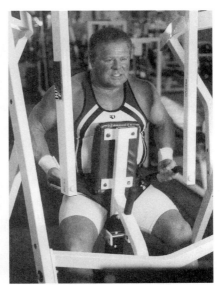

Low Rows

> **LOWER BACK EXERCISES**

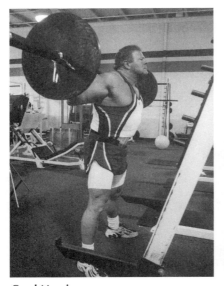

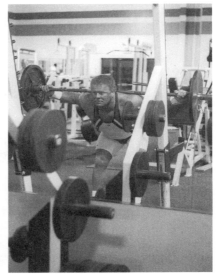

Good Mornings

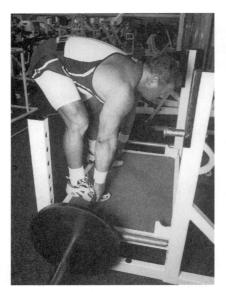

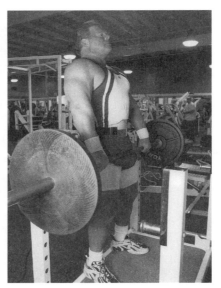

Stiff-Leg Dead Lifts

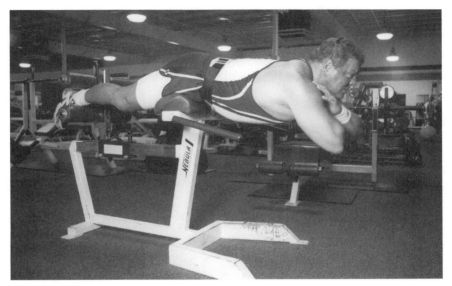

Hyper-Extensions

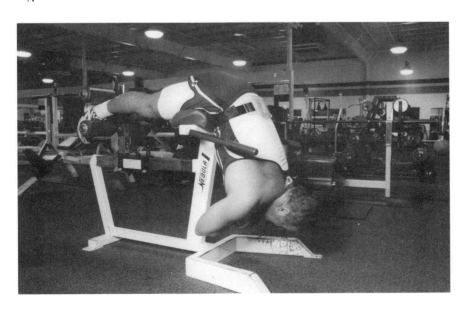

CALORIES BURNED PER 30 MINUTES OF MODERATE EXERCISE

Aerobics (high impact)	252 calories burned
Aerobics (low impact)	171 calories burned
Ballet	177 calories burned
Calisthenics (push-ups, crunches)	236 calories burned
Funk/Hip Hop Classes	183 calories burned
Jumping Rope	295 calories burned
Kickboxing	335 calories burned
Rock Wall Climbing	324 calories burned
Spinning	270 calories burned
Step Aerobics	337 calories burned
Tai Chi	118 calories burned
Water Aerobics	118 calories burned
Yoga	118 calories burned
Backpacking	207 calories burned
Canoeing	103 calories burned
Cross-Country Skiing	236 calories burned
Cycling (12–14 mph)	236 calories burned
Downhill Skiing	148 calories burned
In-Line Skating	207 calories burned
Kayaking	148 calories burned
Mountain Biking	251 calories burned
Power Walking	171 calories burned
Running (easy pace)	266 calories burned
Scuba Diving	207 calories burned
Skateboarding	148 calories burned
Snowboarding	213 calories burned
Snowshoeing	236 calories burned
Trail Walking	144 calories burned
Walking	141 calories burned
Cross-Country Ski Machine	280 calories burned
Rowing Machine	207 calories burned
Stair Climber	177 calories burned
Stationary Biking	310 calories burned
Treadmill Running	369 calories burned
Treadmill Walking (flat, 4.5 mph)	133 calories burned

(continues)

CALORIES BURNED PER 30 MINUTES OF MODERATE EXERCISE

Treadmill Walking (incline, 5.2 mph)	210 calories burned
VersaClimber	322 calories burned
Basketball (just shooting around)	133 calories burned
Beach Volleyball	236 calories burned
Golf	162 calories burned
Martial Arts	295 calories burned
Racquetball	207 calories burned
Swimming	236 calories burned

AN EATING PLAN THAT WILL KEEP THE FAT OFF

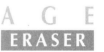

What if the pounds have really crept up on you, and you have a serious problem of 20 to 30 pounds of excess weight? What do you do? The first thing you must do is have a serious talk with yourself and set a realistic goal. If you have allowed yourself to get 30 pounds overweight, one option that desperate people take is to go on a short-term starvation diet that promises to take off 30 pounds in 4 to 6 weeks. Is this possible? Yes it is. Is it *possible* to keep it off? Yes it is. Is it *probable* that you will keep it off? No it is not.

It is unrealistic to believe that you could deplete the fat cells in your body in a six-week period of time, and keep the weight off. After you've gained and lost a lot of weight, your body acts just like a balloon. Once you let all of the air out, it is a lot easier to blow it up the second or third time. People who crash diet often end up putting all of the weight back on and then some. Why is this? Simply because we have to accept that nature is not a bungler. Starting way back in prehistoric times, when our bodies were food deprived for a long period of time, we learned to store fat and to give it up reluctantly.

When you ask your metabolic system to do something it does not want to do and you crash diet, you have thrown its timing clock completely out of line. The first rule of the body is to get back in line, because it wants to be well balanced. So it tries hard to hold onto fat. That is why crash diets are so frequently counterproductive. You must take the weight off in a very sensible and intelligent way. Give yourself ten weeks instead of six. So you'll have to plan your pre-reunion diet a little sooner.

What do I consider a realistic and safe amount of weight to lose weekly? I believe you can lose 5 pounds your very first week. Then 4 pounds the second week, and in the third week, you can safely drop 3 pounds. If you can maintain a 2- to 3-pound loss per week for the next 6 weeks, you will be doing fine and remain healthy. Over a 10-week period of time what would that be? Week 1 = 5 pounds. Week 2 = 4 pounds. Week 3 = 3 pounds. Now you have lost 12 pounds with 7 weeks to go.

If you simply average a 2-pound loss for the next 7 weeks, you will have taken off 26 pounds. If you average 3, then you will have taken off 33 pounds of weight in 10 weeks. Bear in mind that this is not 6 weeks. This is 10 full weeks. This allows your body to get used to the weight loss, your metabolism to become regular, the deprivation cravings to end, and your activity level to increase so that your cardiovascular and respiratory systems learn to handle the increased activity levels without an increase in appetite.

This is a very safe way to take up to 30 pounds off in a 10-week period. I said that my goal was to keep my recommendations simple. It's not complicated, but you need to exhibit the mental toughness to stick with the plan. It is just a fact of metabolic life that the exact places you most want to lose fat are the places that stubbornly resist giving it up. You have to be more persistent than those fat cells.

For 10 weeks you must adhere strictly to the principles I outline in this chapter: Elevated protein; reduced carbohydrate and very limited amounts of fat (the good fats); fat-burning exercise, including resistance training and aerobics; a great deal of water; and a definite detoxification program. It works and keeps your body strong. Most importantly, it helps create an optimum lean muscle mass/body fat ratio.

FOLLOW THESE 6 SIMPLE STEPS TO BENEFIT MOST FROM YOUR NEW EATING PLAN

1. Drink a minimum of ten 12-ounce glasses of pure water per day. I prefer distilled water, because water is only important for hydration. Anything else that you might find in water can be found elsewhere more efficiently. *Note: this is a minimum. If you exercise, you should drink an ounce of water for every pound of body weight.*

2. Determine how many pounds of fat you want to lose. (Notice I didn't say how much *weight* you want to lose.)

3. Design an exercise plan that you will stick with, at least for the duration of the fat-reduction period. Remember to cycle your exercises (see next chapter). Calculate your incremental calorie burn per week.

4. Plan your weekly diet according to the 60 percent protein, 30 percent complex carbohydrates, 10 percent healthy fats combination, or one of the other plans if you are especially active. Use the food table provided at the end of this chapter to calculate the percentage of calories you are getting from each group.

5. Determine the number of calories you will burn with your chosen exercise, and then how many calories you must limit yourself to, in order to create the fat burning you desire. Remember to lose a pound of fat, it takes a 3000-calorie burnoff/calorie-reduction combination.

6. Keep track of your progress weekly. Are you meeting your goals? You need a tape measure handy to track the number of inches you are loosing from those difficult regions. Keep in mind all of those ugly numbers about fat and disease, and keep thinking how great you're going to look and feel at the end of 10 weeks!

FOOL YOUR BODY BY CYCLING YOUR FOODS

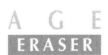

Just as I cycle my exercises to fool my body, I like to take my body through different stages of what is called the SDAF—specific dynamic action of food. This was explained earlier in the chapter when I discussed the body heat required to digest protein, carbohydrates, and fat. Because protein requires a greater heat elevation and a longer digesting period, it is best to eat protein without fat-containing foods or minimize the consumption of foods with high fat grams. This is one of my fat-busting secrets. Break your eating pattern by cycling your food in a three-day eating pattern. This will trick your body into burning more fat.

Here's how cycling your food works:

DAY ONE: Eat your proteins in the morning with little or no fat. The reason for this is that the high protein turns up the metabolic rate by 30 percent. The fat only raises metabolism 4 percent. So for the long hours required to digest the protein, the body is digesting fat and never has the chance to store it. The light fat intake is not enough to create an energy burn, and there are no carbohydrates available to be burned as energy, so stored fat cells must be used for energy.

DAY TWO: Eat your carbohydrates in the morning with minimal amounts of fat, and eat your proteins in the afternoon. On this day, the carbohydrates that are the energy fuel source ignite the body's energy by elevating glucose levels, and since there is no protein, which is so necessary to sustain glucose levels, the body burns the carbohydrates, the minimum fat available, and then again goes to stored fat for energy. The addition of the protein in the afternoon will elevate the metabolism by 30 percent and once again continue to burn any of the unused fats or carbohydrates from breakfast. And then add protein in the evening with light carbohydrates. The protein eaten in the evening again elevates the body temperature by 30 percent, thus sustaining glucose levels while burning the light carbohydrates and calling upon stored fat cells for energy.

DAY THREE: Eat your carbohydrates and fats in the morning, with only light protein. Then at lunchtime eat the balance of your fats, and in the evening eat another load of protein. This energizes the body, increases glucose levels supported by just enough protein to keep your metabolism active for three to four hours. This is a great day to do your most strenuous or active physical workout of the week. For lunch you eat the balance of fats and no carbohydrates. The glucose levels begin to drop and with no protein to support the glucose levels, stored fat once again becomes the provider of energy, increasing fat calorie burn. The increased amount of protein in the evening sustains the high metabolic level, thus burning off any unused fats or carbohydrates from the day. At the same time, the protein provides nutrition to rebuild muscle tissue broken down during exercise.

Using this eating plan moves your body's thermostat up and down, keeping it constantly active. *By cycling your foods, you prevent your body's settling into a rut that will facilitate fat storage. It will remain active and operate at a higher metabolic, fat-burning rate. Get your body's internal system used to having to separate food types.* Never let your body get comfortable dealing with food.

Another technique is to keep your body working at all times with less food. If you eat five or six small "meals" of 200–250 calories, you can trigger the body into thinking "uh-oh, here comes fat," and then it burns it. This process works especially well for women, because a woman's hormone level cycles less frequently than a man's does—every six hours instead of four. The more frequent triggers will help keep the fat-burning process going throughout the day. This keeps your metabolic rate working almost continually during your waking hours.

Now that we've covered how to get rid of the fat you've accumulated over the past several years, the next chapter is going to show you how to gain back that young, lean physique you thought was gone forever. Next summer, I want the beach to be your *friend!*

NUTRITION VALUE OF SOME COMMON FOODS

FOOD	QUANTITY	CALORIES	PROTEIN GRAMS	FAT GRAMS	CARBOHYDRATE GRAMS
Chicken (light meat)	16 oz	753	88	15.4	0
Chicken (dark meat)	16 oz	798	80	28.6	0
Turkey (light meat)	16 oz	798	96	17.7	0
Hamburger 21% fat	16 oz	932	78.9	66.2	0
Tuna (in oil)	7-oz can	570	47.9	40.6	0
Tuna (in water)	7-oz can	251	55.4	1.6	0
Shrimp (boiled)	16 oz	1021	92.1	49.0	45.4
Cheddar Cheese	8 oz	903	32	73.1	4.8
Milk (non-fat)	32 oz	353	40	0	50
Milk (low-fat, 2%)	32 oz	581	36	19.7	59

(continues)

NUTRITION VALUE OF SOME COMMON FOODS

FOOD	QUANTITY	CALORIES	PROTEIN GRAMS	FAT GRAMS	CARBOHYDRATE GRAMS
Butter (1 stick)	4 oz	812	7	91.9	.5
Eggs (chicken)	1 lg.	112	7.2	8.9	.2
Apple	1	123	4	1.3	30.7
Orange	1	64	1.3	.3	16
Peach	1	58	.9	.2	14.8
Pear	1	100	1.1	.7	25.1
Strawberries	1pt.	121	2.3	1.6	27.4
Brown Rice	16 oz	540	11.3	2.7	115.7
Egg Noodles	16 oz	1760	58.1	20.9	326.6
Walnuts	4 oz	210	5	20	3
Bean Sprouts	16 oz	127	14.5	.9	23.6
Brussels Sprouts	16 oz	163	19.1	1.8	29
Cucumber	1	45	2.7	.3	10.2
Lettuce	1 head	70	4.8	.5	15.6
Potato	16 oz	295	8.6	.5	65.8
Corn	16 oz	376	14.5	4.5	85.3
Tomato	1	27	1.4	.2	5.8

four
the secret to restoring your
youthful figure or physique

Doesn't it just bug you when someone begins a sentence with "I hate to have to tell you this, but . . ."? Well, I'm going to be that guy. Please forgive me, but I have to begin by telling you that this chapter, of all the chapters in this book, was the most difficult to write. Why? Because *I hate to have to tell you this, but . . .* the information in this chapter should be a book all by itself. Therefore, this will be a crash course that I hope will help you begin to take control of your body, its cravings, its wants, and its needs. And if I only succeed in getting you up off the couch and into the proper mental attitude, I'll have accomplished what I've set out to do here!

Did you ever look at an old photo of yourself at the beach and wonder what ever happened to that lean, firm, youthful figure of yours? Face it, for a great majority of us, what takes place during that 10-year span between 24 and 34, or between 34 and 44, doesn't do wonders for our confidence at swimsuit time. Don't you just hate it when your kids squeeze that pudge hanging over the too-tight elastic band on your swimsuit and screech with laughter, "Dad, what is this?" Or when you realize that the "baby" you're blaming for the tummy sticking out over your bikini bottom is 15 years old?

In this chapter, I'm going to take you through a system of total body exercises that will bring back the tone and shape that made you feel good about yourself over a decade ago. Remember the shape that you had before the years of 12-hour workdays spent juggling careers and parenthood, power breakfasts, lunches on the run, dinner meetings, fast food eaten in the car while driving your kids to Little League and piano lessons took their toll? Remember that pre-childbirth waistline that you now accommodate with elastic waistbands? And what about the results of weekends in front of the television with beer and the popcorn bowl?

As I stated in an earlier chapter, the average baby boomer experiences a 14-percent decline in lean muscle mass between the ages of 25 and 35. And if that's not bad enough, another 14 percent of muscle is lost between the ages of 35 and 45. That's nearly one-third less muscle in only 20 years! And this applies especially to women, who, because of their hormonal makeup, have less muscle mass to begin with. My goal here is to see to it that you reverse that downward spiral and build your muscle mass back to where it was 10 to 20 years ago.

If you haven't reached your 50s or 60s yet, I apologize for being the bearer of bad news, but, on average, muscle loss in this phase of life is even more dramatically severe. However, I wouldn't dream of bringing you bad tidings without offering some very good news to offset it. That's what this chapter is all about. It's devoted to helping you regain your lean muscle mass at whatever age you have decided to make a lifestyle change. And I will not ask you to live in the gym to accomplish this goal. As you read on you might challenge this last statement, thinking you'll never be able to find the time to do what I ask. However, with practice you'll quickly learn to make economical and efficient use of your exercise time. You'll feel so much better that everything you do will be done faster and *more effectively*. And think about this: If you work an average 40-hour week and sleep 55 to 60 hours of that week, you still have 68 hours left. I'm asking for 10 to 12 of those hours each week to completely change your life.

I am very confident that if you give me just three days a week for ten weeks (and maybe a few more days in the last week), I can give you back the figure or physique that you know is the *real* you. If you're interested in a more athletic physique, I'll offer you a six-day-a-week program. If you are a willing student, I will be your coach and long-distance personal trainer, helping you achieve the shape you desire.

Although I am obviously writing this book from a male perspective, I have spent a great portion of my adult life in the health spa industry working primarily with women. Thirty years ago I saw women spending most of their gym or spa time on the old-fashioned roller machines or vibrating belts that were supposed to roll the fat off your thighs and shake your waist to a smaller size. Or, they would spend their time pedaling a stationary bike or trying to sweat off fat in the steam room.

Without changing their eating habits or increasing their lean muscle mass, these women wondered why it was so hard to lose weight or regain their figure. Much of this thought process can be blamed on the state of exercise science as it related to women at that time. It has only been in the last 10 to 15 years that we have exploded those old myths and learned, through exhaustive research, the many benefits of lean muscle mass to the female body.

Over the years it has been my experience that most men almost naturally want to "pump iron" in one form or another. Many remember the first time they heard the story of Charles Atlas having sand kicked in his face by a bully at the beach, and deciding to do something about it. They too want to be strong enough to face down the bully. My own personal life in fitness started at age 11, when I picked up my first weight and attempted to do a set of curls. My only goal at that time was to have bigger biceps—to show off in my tight T-shirts. I think I too had seen one too many of those Charles Atlas ads on the back pages of my comic books! But soon the improvement that the weight training made in my overall athletic prowess, and in my ability to perform in all of my chosen sports, provided the inspiration for my lifetime commitment to fitness.

In the years that followed, I became very serious about Olympic-style weight lifting. By age 17, I was the youngest participant in the national qualifying finals of the Pan Am Games. Even though I eventually lost the competition, this experience gave me a sense of pride and a commitment that led me to want to excel in everything I was ever going to do.

While assisting in building one of the largest health club chains in the world, I was directly involved in the opening or supervision of 59 separate health spas throughout the United States. I truly believe that during those 17 years I helped thousands of people not only build better bodies, but I also helped increase their overall zest for living. It was during these years that women and their budding interest in weight-training activities dictated to me that I had to broaden my education to include the particular needs of female weight training.

It was once believed that as a man lifted weights he got larger, bulging muscles that would slow him down and impede his flexibility and coordination. We now know that without weight training, it is impossible to compete successfully at higher athletic levels. Not only does weight training not impede speed, flexibility, and coordination, it does the exact opposite.

When I first had the opportunity to introduce weight training into the sport of major league baseball, it became one of the more controversial times of my life. In the mid-1970s the hierarchy that was running the game were naysayers when it came to weight training. They believed it would make the players muscle-bound and slow them down. They believed that it would slow their running speed, their bat speed, and that it would interfere with their fluid throwing motion. Not only was this an inaccurate analysis of the effect of weight training on their bodies, in fact, the exact opposite was true here too.

The athletes became bigger, stronger, faster, and more fluid and graceful in their motions. Bat speed increased, more power pitchers were developed, and the offensive explosion in baseball began. There are those who would tell you that it is a "juiced up" baseball that has led to all the home runs. I'm telling you to look into the weight-training facilities provided in every locker room and spring-training facility in baseball. Or look at the definition in players' backs or the size of their forearms and upper arms, and you will know where this offensive explosion in baseball is coming from. Tell Mark McGwire and his 98-mile-per-hour bat speed that weight training is slowing him down.

Through weight training, my program helped elevate the performance of all-star players like Nolan Ryan, Ozzie Smith, Dave Parker, Don Baylor, Lance Parrish, Brian Downing, and more. Through my friend Joe Morgan, my weight-training program helped the entire Oakland Athletics team the year that they brought up a skinny rookie named Mark McGwire. Not only did my program help increase their power, but it also helped to extend their careers, leading them to increased earning power and greater financial stability for the rest of their lives.

A few years later, through my friend Dr. Ernie Vandeweghe, my program helped the Los Angeles Lakers championship team of the 1980s in the same capacity. If you compare photos of today's players with those in earlier years, you'll see that the biggest difference, other than the tight shorts they used to wear, is the muscular development and powerful physiques that almost every NBA player has today.

And now look at the fruits of weight training beginning to make their impact in women's sports. Women golfers come to the PGA training center in Palm Beach, Florida, to improve all aspects of their game. In the world of tennis, the Williams sisters—Venus and Serena—have ridden their strength training to center court at Wimbledon. A more mature and muscularly developed Jennifer Capriati won her first grand slam in 2001.

Perhaps the most important exercise/fitness concept to come out of the last decade or so is the undeniable fact that women, not just men, also increase their speed, stamina, endurance, flexibility, overall athletic ability, and general well-being with weight training. *And it has not been at the cost of their femininity.*

When I enter gyms, health clubs, spas, and fitness centers today, I see women curling dumbbells, bench-pressing, doing squats and leg extensions, and participating in all forms of weight training. These women are among the growing number who have discovered the enormous benefits of the combination of weight training and aerobic activity to their vitality and quality of life. And no, they don't all have bulging biceps, rippling thighs, and big broad backs. The relatively few women who look that way are usually found in extreme competitions and may also exhibit masculine features and other secondary male characteristics.

None of this overdevelopment in women has anything to do with simply lifting weights. These women have chosen to use steroids or other legal or illegal substances and will sooner or later pay a price for their choice. The fact is, women can only increase in muscle mass to the degree that their *naturally* occurring female hormones will allow. Women simply do not have the hormones necessary to match the muscle growth of men. Please don't let anyone tell you otherwise.

Weight training increases lean muscle mass. Increased lean muscle mass causes a constant increase in metabolic rate. Just a slight increase in muscle mass and metabolic rate causes an enormous increase in the amount of fat burned while training or doing aerobic exercise. So while women can and should certainly continue doing aerobic exercise to stay slim and burn fat, there is no denying that including weight training in an overall exercise plan can help them reach their goal even faster, *no matter what their age.*

Over the last three years, I have enjoyed working with the women who compete in what are called tri-fitness competitions. These are not the grotesquely overdeveloped women you see in extreme weight-lifting competitions. They are women like Tanya Merryman and Katie Uter, who have developed their fitness program to include just enough aerobic exercise and weight training. These women are feminine, shapely, muscular, strong, and beautiful. They have careers and many of them are mothers. They are living proof of what the right fitness regimen can produce.

Do you think I am placing too much emphasis on weight training? If you think I am, or if you think I am "overselling" the concept, I will tell you I don't think that's possible when it comes to age management and a Forever Young lifestyle.

A very well documented study at Tufts University proved that *even men and women over the age of 85* who began using weights in load-bearing exercises increased both their muscle power and stamina. Men over 85 even increased their muscle size and density. Greater muscle power provides greater joint and bone support, and thus helps fight osteoporosis—a problem now documented not just in aging females, but in aging males, as well.

Think of that! The individuals in this study were in their ninth decade of life and still made positive and documented changes in their quality of life—because they trained with weights. So, no, I don't think I can overemphasize the importance I place on weight training in age management.

NOURISH YOUR MUSCLES

If you want to build your muscles, you have to nourish them through your bloodstream. This is why I've previously recommended a high-protein diet involving consumption of 60 percent protein, 30 percent carbohydrates, and 10 percent fat. In addition to protein-rich foods, I supplement my diet with protein powders that help my body create enough nitrogen to repair the muscle tissue I break down by exercising.

Your cardiovascular system sends fuel and food throughout your body, especially into the areas in your body that you are working. It is just as necessary to assist your cardiovascular system with adequate vitamins and minerals. I add additional herbs to my diet as adaptogens, and large dosages of antioxidants. Excessive amounts of exercise will also produce an excessive amount of free radicals in the system, which must be fought and removed. If you want to get the maximum from each workout, don't starve your muscles with inadequate diet or lack of food supplementation.

People who go on diets without supplementation and then spend hours in the gym are wasting their time because they are severely limiting their body's ability to build calorie-burning muscle mass and to recover completely. I stay away from any type of artificial stimulant that contains ma huang or ephedrine. It goes without saying that steroids are completely off the chart.

I used to consume literally handfuls of vitamins, in doses way over the recommended amount, because I know that the hydrochloric acid in our stomachs destroy almost all of the nutrients contained in most vitamins. Since the stomach and hydrochloric acid destroy most of the nutrients in these food supplements *before* they can get to the cellular/molecular level, I had to overload in order to get the minimums I needed.

To this end, I collaborated with several leading pharmacologists, who helped develop a series of molecules in a linear chain that escort the necessary nutrients through the acid-filled digestive tract and, like a missile warhead, send them through the bloodstream to hook up directly at the cellular/molecular level. We created an age- and pain-management product to fulfill necessary balanced nutritional needs. This new product supplies each nutrient in proper balance—vitamins, minerals, herbs, and state-of-the-art growth factor peptides. It comes in a crystalline effervescent form that dissolves in water, producing a pleasant-tasting drink. Like a mini–heat shield, the escort molecule protects the nutrients through the stomach, providing three to five times the bioavailability of any nutritional tablet, caplet, or capsule. The nutrients are delivered at the cellular level with all of their power and full activity level still in force. (See the reference section if you would like more information about this age-management product.)

You may be using products that you believe can supply your body with some of the same nutrients. The important thing is to give the tissue in your muscles the optimum environment for growing and building.

Because of my belief in the importance of providing oxygenation and nourishment to the muscles, we created another product called MaxEndorphin Plus. This isn't intended to be a sales presentation, but I would be remiss if I didn't briefly tell you about it. The product maximizes your muscle's strength and energy output by oxygenating your muscles, replacing electrolytes, eliminating lactic acid buildup, and speeding recovery. Taken 30 minutes before exercising or engaging in any activity that requires energy, intensity, or mental acuity, MaxEndorphin Plus rushes safe, healthy nutrients into your bloodstream. It is not a steroid. It is not a thermogenic, and it is not an artificial stimulant.

The "Plus" is contained in two nutrients that help you after your activity. One is D-ribose, which promotes recovery and muscle growth in as little as 12 to 24 hours. The other is glutamine for tissue repair. Glutamine is an amino acid that prevents muscles from entering a catabolic state during physical activity. This allows for faster muscle growth and a significant reduction in body fat. If you want to learn more about MaxEndorphin Plus, see the reference section or log on to **BillFranks ForeverYoung.com.**

AGE ERASER

CYCLE YOUR EXERCISES

I am a great believer in cycling your exercises. What does this mean? Exactly what it sounds like. You must regularly change your workout, modifying every aspect of what you do. You must cycle various types of exercises, the number of repetitions, the degree of intensity, and the amount of weight used. This applies to weight-lifting routines, but it also applies to any aerobic program you may use.

If you want a rapid improvement in the shape of your body, don't let your body get comfortable in any routine. If it gets comfortable and if it gets used to the workload and the output of energy required, *the muscular gain will be drastically reduced.* As soon as your body learns to handle a task with relative ease, it will kick back, relax, and stop making progress. You reach a level that is very difficult to improve upon. In weight training, we call this the *plateau.* You try to pull out of it, but it seems like you are endlessly stuck. It feels like you're on a treadmill getting nowhere. Runners call this "hitting the wall" and they too must find ways to trick their body into reaching the next level.

I get hundreds of letters and e-mails each year from people who can't seem to make progress, even though they say that they are working harder and longer, and sweating more than ever before. In a majority of cases, they are telling the truth. The problem is that they are not working *smarter.* I want you to work smarter. You'll be able to cut down the time that you put in at the gym, or wherever you participate in your exercise regime, while increasing your benefits. And you'll also give yourself more time to enjoy these benefits.

People who have hit the plateau have entered what their body considers a comfort zone. Their bodies are not being put into overload where additional muscle strength or cardiovascular stamina is required to increase the forward movement. As a result, they are treading water and are not where they want to be.

I devote myself to some form of exercise between four to six days per week (more than you need to do to complete this program). But you must understand that this my life. I don't know what it feels like to live a life that some may consider normal. I don't feel I would be as qualified to write this book if I hadn't attempted to push the envelope in the area of fitness. I push myself to experiment and experience the difference between what might be considered normal, and what I consider might be the *normal* of a highly active individual.

I change my exercise routine every three weeks—no exception to this rule. I plan my routines six and nine weeks out. And even if I miss a day of exercise (which occasionally happens, no matter how hard you try to be faithful), I still switch my program at the end of each three-week period. I am specifically speaking now to those of you who want to use weight training combined with cardiovascular training to cycle this great miracle called your body.

Built into my four to six times per week cycle are at least three days that include aerobic training. Aerobics balance off the increase of muscle density provided by weight training, with the added benefits of increased oxygenation, cardiovascular flow, and fat burning. I personally choose cross-training devices for my cardio work; you are free to choose any type you wish.

There are literally hundreds of variations of exercises for your body. The more you learn about your body—and you will definitely learn more as time goes by—you and you alone will determine which of these groups of exercises give you maximum benefit. On pages 58–60 I demonstrate some examples of specific exercises, but I recommend Bill Pearl's book, *Keys to the Kingdom*, which can provide you with multiple examples of exercise groupings to choose from as you switch your routines around.

The important thing to remember here is not so much what exercise you choose to do for each body part, but the cycling of these exercises and the method used in training combinations and variations of repetitions and weight levels. If you follow this plan, your body will never get used to what you are doing. It will constantly have to make adjustments to increase strength and to adjust to the constant changing of your internal organs. And as the muscle tissue works harder, it breaks down, separates, and regenerates, coming back bigger and stronger, with far more density and in far better condition.

The great side benefit to all of this is that the increase in muscle mass will cause a continually elevated metabolic rate that will increase the fat-burning ability of your body. This, in turn, will lower the level of bad LDL (low-density lipid fat) cholesterol and increase the level of good HDL (high-density lipid fat) cholesterol. Proper levels of LDL and HDL must be maintained to reduce the risk of coronary problems. Remember, it's mind over muscle matter, so let's start cycling!

PUSH AND PULL YOURSELF INTO SHAPE

If you want maximum results from your weight-training program, you should alternate push and pull days in your workout. What is the *push-pull* theory? The push is chest, triceps (back of arms), and deltoids—or the shoulder region—because you are usually pushing the weight away from you. The pull exercises, also called contractile exercises, are those that pull the weight back toward your body. They are, for the most part, the back and the biceps (front of the arms). Leg extensions are open, or pulled, while squats are push exercises. You will note that I designed the cycled routines based on these principles. One day you push, the next day you pull.

The push-pull technique is so important because of the physiological process of building muscle mass. It is actually *after* the workout, in the recovery or anabolic state, that new muscle mass is generated. By following the push-pull method, while you are busy working on a new muscle group, your body is still busy building muscle from your previous workout. This allows for the recovery of the push muscles while you are working on the pull and vice versa. Once you and your body figure out how to work together, you will be amazed at how quickly you will progress.

On push days, I do cardiovascular work. I spend 45 minutes on my treadmill—walking the first 10 minutes at 3.5 miles per hour, then jogging at 5.5 miles per hour for 5 or 6 minutes, then walking for another 4 or 5 minutes at 4.5 miles per hour. I finish up for another 10 minutes at a 6.5-miles-per-hour jog, and the balance of time will be spent at a low-intensity walking pace at anywhere from 3.8 to 4.5 miles per hour. I'm describing my schedule in such specific detail as an example of, and to emphasize, how I vary each aspect of my workout, *whether it involves weights or aerobics*. By doing 45 minutes of treadmill, I also gain some fat-burning results.

You need to determine what amount of time and intensity level is

WEEK 1

On the first 3 days, using dumbbells and machines, do 2–3 exercises per body part with 3–4 sets of 12–15 repetitions for each exercise you choose.

DAY 1: Work your chest, shoulders, and triceps (back of upper arm). Follow with 30 minutes of aerobic/cardiovascular exercise.

DAY 2: Work your back, biceps (front of upper arm), abdomen, and forearms.

DAY 3: Work your legs including quadriceps (front of the thigh), hamstrings, and calves.

Follow your leg workout with 12–18 minutes of low-intensity aerobic/cardiovascular exercise to recirculate your blood.

On days 4–6, using barbells and machines, do 2–3 exercises per body part with 3–4 sets of 10–12 repetitions for each exercise you choose.

DAY 4: Again, work your chest, shoulders, and triceps.

DAY 5: Again, work your back, biceps, abdomen, and forearms. Follow this with 45 minutes of aerobics/cardiovascular exercise.

DAY 6: Again, work your legs including quadriceps, hamstrings, and calves.

WEEK 2

Week 2 is the same as week 1 except for the number of sets and repetitions. On days 1–3, do 3–4 sets and 10–12 repetitions of each exercise. On days 4–6, do 3–4 sets and 8–10 repetitions of each exercise. This will allow you to increase the amount of weight you lift if that is what you desire.

WEEK 3

This week we change the order of body parts. On the first 3 days of this week, work with heavy weights. Do 2–3 exercises per body part, with 3–4 sets and 6 repetitions of each exercise.

DAY 1: Work your legs, including quadriceps, hamstrings, and calves. Follow with 12–15 minutes of aerobic/cardiovascular work.

CYCLE 1 (CONTINUED)

DAY 2: Work your chest, shoulders, and triceps. Follow with 30 minutes of aerobic/cardiovascular work.

DAY 3: Work your back, biceps, abdomen, and forearms. Follow with 45 minutes of aerobic/cardiovascular work.

Repeat the same body parts on days 4–6. Work even heavier—to approximately 80 percent of your maximum power. Do only 4–6 repetitions of each exercise.

CYCLE 2

Repeat all 3 weeks of cycle 1, *using completely different exercises*. Work the body parts in the same sequence you did in cycle 1. However, choose a different exercise or change the sequence of the exercises. For example, although you will continue to work your chest, shoulders, and triceps, either reverse the order of exercises or change to different exercises, so that your muscles get a little different communication from your brain.

CYCLE 3

This is the power cycle. Repeat all 3 weeks of cycle 2, *again using completely different exercises*. Choose 3 exercises per body part. Work heavy and do only 4–6 repetitions the first 3 days of the week, and just 4 repetitions the last 3 days of the week. To help rid yourself of the lactic acid buildup during this cycle, include at least one 20-minute and two 45-minute aerobic/cardiovascular sessions each week. This will also increase the blood flow to all of your muscle tissue, allowing your system to recover from this heavy overload.

best for you. Start slow and build. Small successes mean complete victory. If you rush yourself to levels of discomfort, you'll likely quit and then nothing will be accomplished. On pages 63–78 are some of my recommendations for exercises. You may use them or choose your own. Either way, begin *now!*

TEN WEEKS TO A FOREVER YOUNG FIGURE

You may not have 6 days each week to build your program. You may decide that you want to do it in 3 days, which is okay, if you'll also give me 45 minutes on a fourth day for some light aerobics. When you visualize the muscle mass that you will be retrieving from your body's lost and found in just 10 weeks, I know you'll agree it's worth an hour of hard work 3 days a week and some light work on the fourth. If you choose a 3-day-a-week workout program, you should work each muscle group a little longer and a little harder doing a *minimum of 5 sets of 10–12 reps for each body part.* Following is a program that works in 3-week intervals. The tenth week sculpts your body's wonderful finishing touches.

WEEKS 1–3
During your first 3 weeks, do 3 exercises per body part.

DAY 1: Work your chest, shoulders, triceps, and abdominals. Also do some cardiovascular work.

DAY 2: Do your pull exercises: back, biceps, forearms, and abdominals.

DAY 3: Work your legs really, really well. Do another cardiovascular activity all by itself. Either go for a long bike ride or a jog on the treadmill, cross-trainer, or stairclimber—anything that you can do for 45 minutes to an hour.

WEEKS 4–6
During your second 3 weeks, do 2 exercises per body part.

DAY 1: Work your *entire* upper body and do your cardiovascular work.

DAY 2: Work your legs and add abdominal work to the routine.

DAY 3: Do the upper body again—the push, the pull, and the abdominals again. Then call it a day.

DAY 4: Do your cardiovascular/aerobic routine. You're two-thirds of the way home!

WEEKS **7–9**

During your third 3 weeks, do 2 exercises per body part.

DAY 1: Put in 1 hour of cardiovascular work.

DAY 2: Work your legs hard—really hard.

DAY 3: Do your cardiovascular work again, all by itself.

DAY 4: Work your entire upper body. Work it hard. Do 5 sets each of 3 exercises per body part.

DAY 4: Do just cardiovascular/aerobic work.

DAY 5: Come back and work your legs again—really, really hard.

You will now begin to see a muscular, lean, body and you will have cut a lot of fat, especially if you accompanied this program with my basic 60/30/10 diet recommendations from Chapter Three. You will begin to see and feel the trim muscular figure you had when you were a young man or woman. This completes your ninth week.

WEEK **10**

I promised to make your physique or figure the envy of the neighborhood by week 10, so I'm going to ask you to give me a little more during this final week. I want you to work out for 6 days this week. During this last week, make the workouts really short, using one exercise per body part.

DAY 1: Work your chest and do 20 minutes of cardiovascular.

DAY 2: Work your back. Do not work anything else.

DAY 3: Work your shoulders and do your ab work.

DAY 4: Do only your arms.

DAY 5: Work those legs hard.

DAY 6: Do your cardiovascular routine.

➤ CHEST EXERCISES

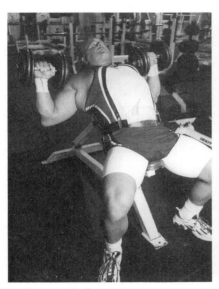 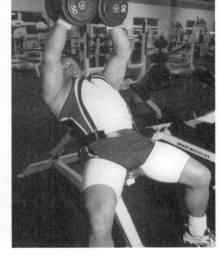

Incline Dumbbell Press

➤ CHEST EXERCISES (CONTINUED)

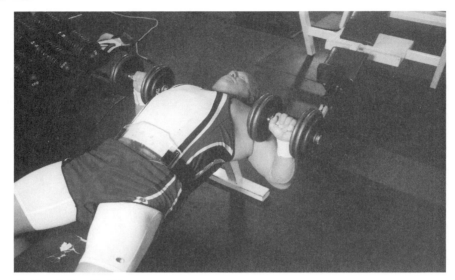

Flat Bench Dumbbell Press

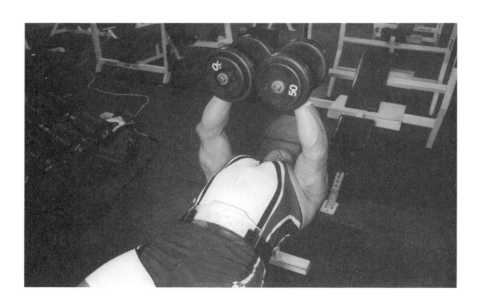

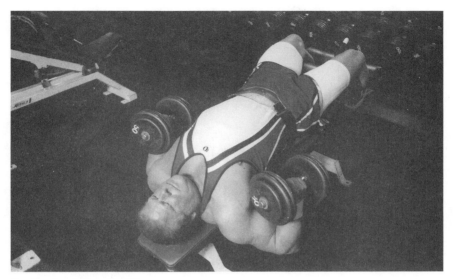

Decline Bench Dumbbell Press

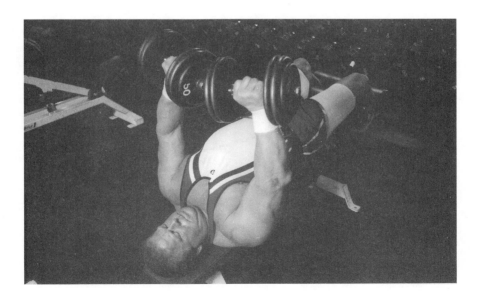

> ### SHOULDER EXERCISES

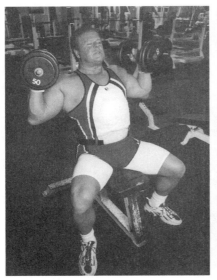 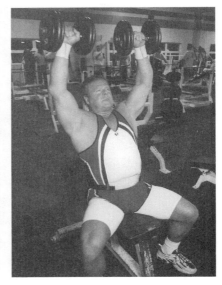

Seated Dumbbell Press

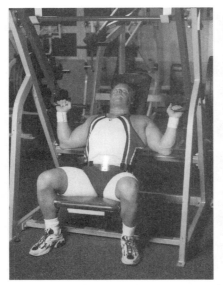 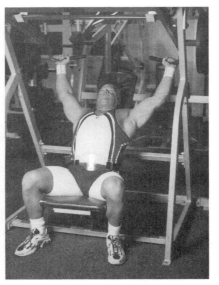

Behind the Neck Press (Using Hammer Machine)

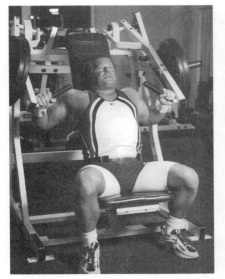 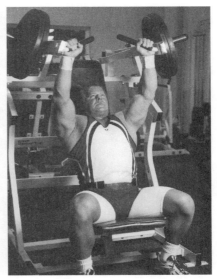

Front Shoulder Press (Using Hammer Machine)

➤ **SHOULDER EXERCISES (CONTINUED)**

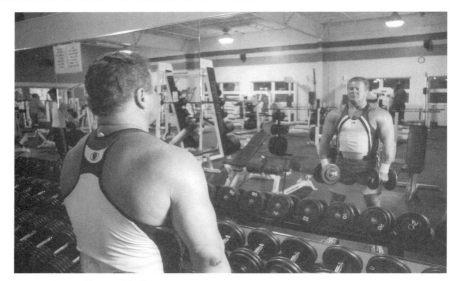

Front Raises with Dumbbells

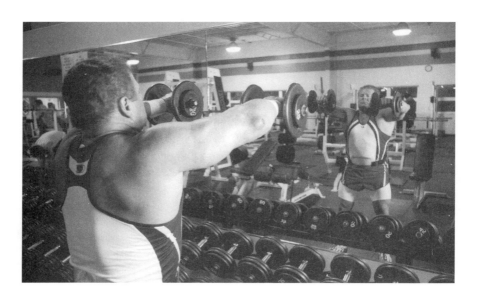

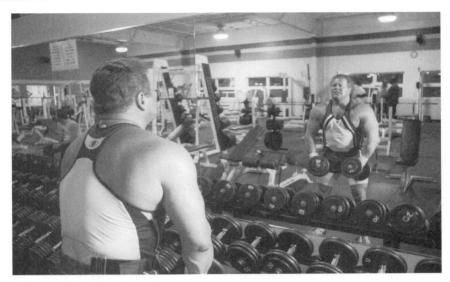

Side Lat Raises with Dumbbells

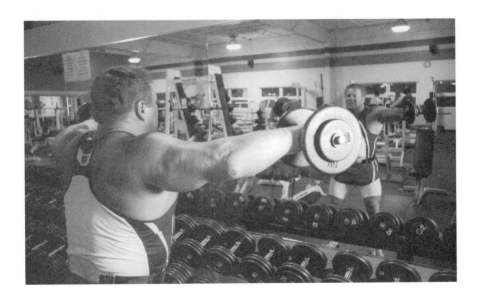

➤ TRICEP EXERCISES

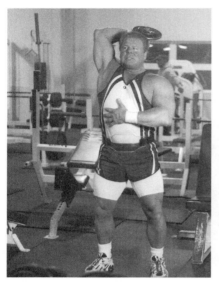 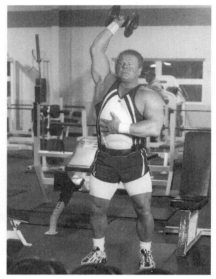

One-Arm Dumbbell Extensions (Do Both Arms!)

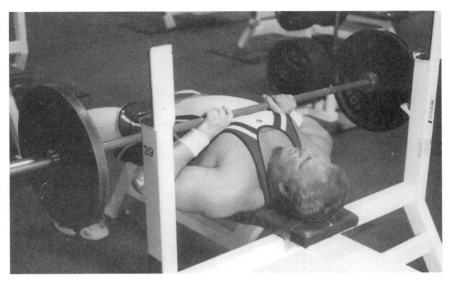

Close-Grip Bench Press

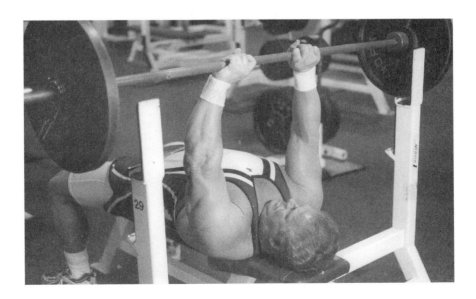

➤ TRICEP EXERCISES (CONTINUED)

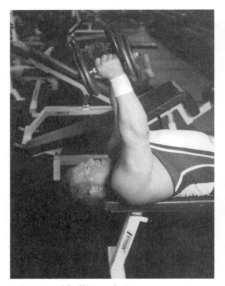 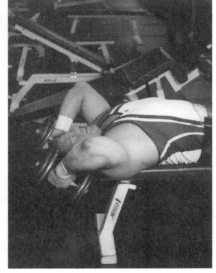

Lying Dumbbell French Press

➤ BACK EXERCISES

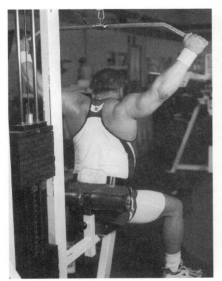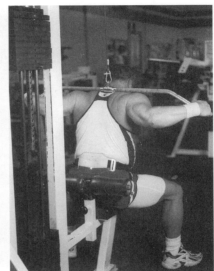

Rear Lat Pull-Downs

➤ **BACK EXERCISES (CONTINUED)**

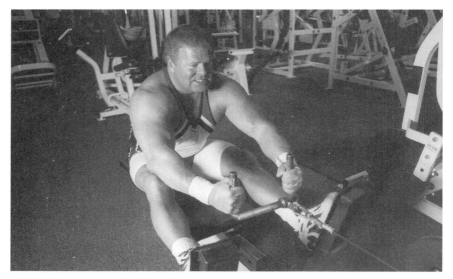

Cable Machine Long Pulls

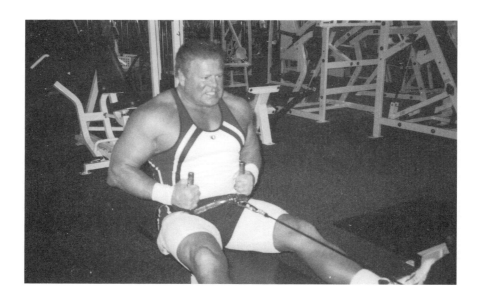

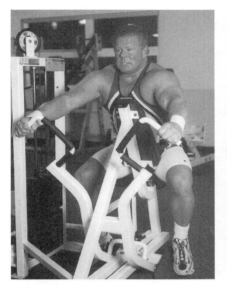
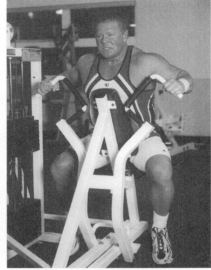

Hammer Machine Rows

➤ BICEP EXERCISES

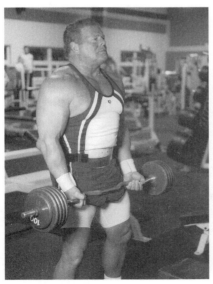
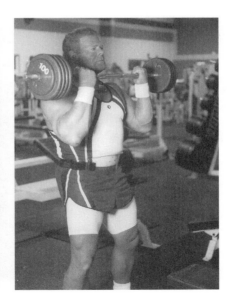

Standing EZ Bar Curls

> ### BICEP EXERCISES (CONTINUED)

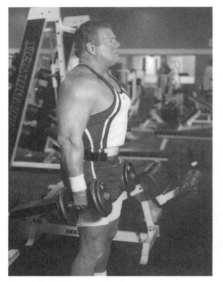

Dumbbell Hammer Curls

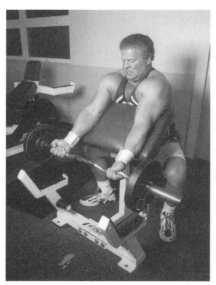

Preacher Bench EZ Bar Curls

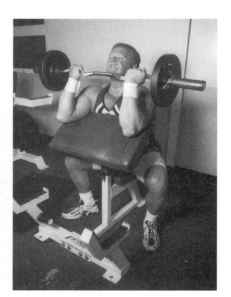

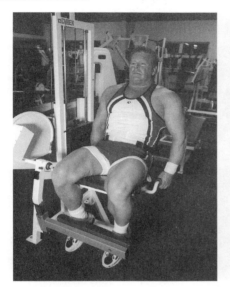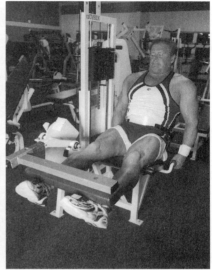

Leg Extensions

➤ **LEG EXERCISES (CONTINUED)**

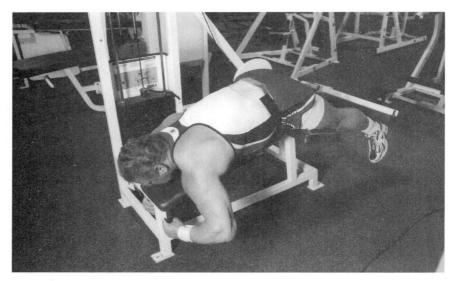

Leg Curls

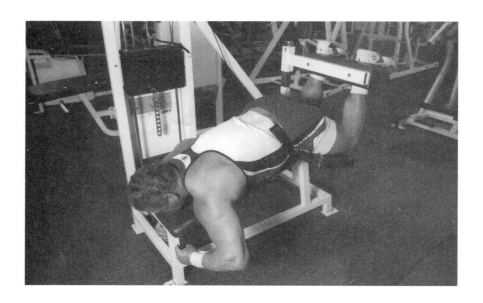

TAKE OFF YOUR CLOTHES AND POSE!

DAY 7: Play Adonis or Venus and stand in front of the mirror or take a picture and compare it to how you looked at the start of the 10 weeks. If you're as happy as I think you will be, give me a call and tell me about it. Send me photos of your transformation and tell me your story. I may call you back and ask you to share your story on my TV show or in my next book.

Nothing makes me happier than people who get to experience the wonderful feeling of reaching their fitness goals and achieving the kind of good health they always knew they were capable of achieving. Do you want to know what's really exciting? Once you achieve this level of accomplishment, you won't want to stop. This is only the beginning of what you can achieve toward better age management and good health. Now you are motivated and excited and full of enthusiasm to learn and do even more!

As you know, I think of myself as your age-management coach, so I'm going to quote another famous coach who mirrors my attitude. It was recently reported that super-coach Phil Jackson once had a talk with his former boss, Jerry Reinsdorf, the owner of the Chicago Bulls. Mr. Reinsdorf asked Phil, "What do you think motivates men, Phil? I think it's greed and fear." Phil responded, "I disagree, Jerry. I think it's love and pride."

I'm with Phil. I know that you are going to be proud of your accomplishment—very proud. And I know that the man or woman you love is going to be ecstatic with the gift that you have given them.

I've trained thousands of people in my life, and this is the moment that makes it all worthwhile. It's a personal triumph and a wonderful feeling when you take control of a very important part of your life. If you're like nearly every single one of the people I've had the pleasure of working with, I know what you want now: *You want more.* You want to get better. You want to get stronger. You want to get more fit. And you want to feel younger. I agree. This is just the beginning of what we can accomplish together.

Now, my friends, I'm sure you understand why I opened this chapter with an apology. As you can now see, an entire book complete with many photos and illustrations could be written about how to perform exercises, breathe properly, and rest adequately in between. I've tried to give you the basic information to get you started.

My job in this chapter was to get you to the point where you can take complete control of your own health and aging. Then, you'll no longer need me as a coach. So keep reading, and let's climb some more mountains and have some more fun!

five

how to save your skin

Right or wrong, your first impression of someone is usually influenced by his or her facial appearance. All of us tend to view someone's face as an age indicator. And whether we want to admit it or not, our satisfaction with our personal appearance, and how others see us, is an important part of our psychological makeup. It is a part of age management that I have always put right up there in importance.

As a newlywed, my wife was somewhat startled to discover that I used more skin-care products than she did! And remember, this was way before all of the cosmetic companies realized that men were an untapped market—a market that just might be interested in keeping their skin young and healthy looking.

Today, of course, there are hundreds of skin-care items packaged for, and marketed to, men. If you read the labels carefully, you will discover that many of the formulas, though packaged as gender specific, are simply the same products in two different containers. However, cosmetic manufacturers still produce a larger variety of products for women, and I still keep buying and experimenting with most of them, regardless of their intended market.

I am frequently asked about my youthful appearance. As you read this, I am 60 years old and have never had any facial cosmetic surgery—not that I have anything against it. I believe surgical corrections and repairs are certainly an option, and I may avail myself of that option sometime in the future. To this point, however, I have been able to maintain the appearance of my skin, not with plastic surgery, but by practicing the skin-care regime I am about to share with you.

Experimenting with cosmetics can become an expensive proposition, but there are many less costly ways to keep your skin healthy and fresh looking. I'll tell you about my skin-care regime, and also tell you about other options that are available.

Most of my suggested age erasers for skin are fairly inexpensive and can be used anywhere your work or play takes you. Others, like cosmetic surgery, require an investment of time and money that you may or may not wish to consider at some point.

My objective here, just as in my television show *Forever Young*, is to make you aware of what's available and what you can reasonably expect if you decide to take advantage of any of these options.

A G E ERASER

DRINK DISTILLED WATER EVERY DAY

The first, one of the most important, and certainly the easiest way to help maintain a youthful appearance is to hydrate your skin—from within. In many chapters of this book you will see that I emphasize the importance of water consumption. I can't say this too many times! You *must* drink water. Your body *craves* it. Your skin *thrives* on it.

I prefer to drink distilled water and I recommend that you do the same. The process of distilling water causes it to become a conduit for the removal of toxins and wastes taken into your body from other foods. Distilled water literally becomes a magnet. It attracts toxins present in your system, and then carries them out of your body when you eliminate. Most normal tap water literally contributes *more* toxins to your body.

Because I work out, I drink one ounce of distilled water for every pound of body weight, *every day*. If you work out or exercise at all, you should do the same. At minimum, you should consume one-half ounce of water for every pound of body weight you carry. For example, if you're a 180-pound man who works out, you should drink 180 ounces of water a day, and 90 ounces a day if you don't work out. A 140-pound woman who works out should drink 140 ounces and at least 70 ounces if she's not exercising.

It's not that tough to do. Once you establish the habit of drinking water all through your day, you'll find that the more you drink, the more you'll crave. And even on the days you don't participate in any formal type of exercise, drinking the amount of water I recommend will keep your body eliminating the toxic wastes that contribute to the aging process.

EXERCISE YOUR SKIN

Exercise is great for your whole body, and this includes your skin, the largest organ of your body. Exercising facial muscles promotes good circulation and good muscle tone. Don't be afraid to stretch the skin of your face. Stretching movements allow your skin to expand and contract, which makes it firmer.

Simple repeated movements like sticking out your tongue as far as it will go and then bringing it back into your mouth, moving your jaw from side to side, moving your eyes in a continual circular motion, sticking out your chin and lower lip, and moving your jaw up and down, may look silly to you, but will strengthen and tone face and neck muscles. And don't be afraid to gently massage your face and neck. Use a light moisturizer or massage lotion so your hands move smoothly and freely over your skin. Move gently around your eyes, and use an upward motion on your neck. This will stimulate circulation and give you a healthy glow.

There is a misconception that exercising your facial muscles may contribute to drooping and sagging. This is just not so. I don't know of anyone who exercises his or her facial muscles any more than actor Jim Carrey. Look closely the next time you watch one of his movies. His facial twists and contortions have not only made him a millionaire, but have contributed to a very youthful appearance.

Your face is no different than any other part of your body. It needs and will respond positively to exercise. So if you're too shy to act like Jim Carrey in public, do your facial exercises in the privacy of your own home. No one will see anything but the positive results.

PRACTICE SMILING OVER FROWNING

The next time you see someone with a gloom-and-doom expression on their face, say something funny and watch how their face changes. I guarantee they will look years younger the moment they smile. A friendly, smiling countenance *looks* younger and makes the person smiling *feel* younger. It also makes those who see a smiling face feel good too!

Put a smile in your voice too. I can't seem to get through a workday without listening to someone's voicemail or answering machine message. I can always tell when someone has recorded a message while smiling—and it makes me want to smile too! Notice how you feel when a smiling, happy person has obviously recorded a message you hear. You don't even have to *see* the face to feel better—and look younger.

So, before you get to the more complex procedures, start with the simplest. Like the song says, "put on a happy face." It is one of the little secrets of people whose skin is described by others as "radiant."

STAND ON YOUR HEAD

Gravity is constantly exerting its force on your body, contributing to the sagging of skin and body parts. I fight this by spending a few minutes upside down every day. Along with all the usual gym equipment, I have always owned a device called a porta-yoga. It's a small padded stool with a cutout, which allows your shoulders to rest on the cushioned portion enabling you to comfortably stand on your head.

But you don't have to have any special equipment to do this. All you need is a clear bit of wall space (remove your shoes so you don't leave marks on the wall), and someone to help you with your first few attempts. Start by standing on your head only 15 to 20 seconds a day and work up to a few minutes every day. Have your helper assist you into position against the wall, holding your legs in place if necessary. Ask them to stay and help you bring your feet back down again. Use a helper until you're comfortable doing it on your own without assistance.

After a few days of practice you will be able to stand on your head quickly, and it won't be long before you begin to see the positive results of reversing the negative effects of gravity. The increase of blood and oxygen has an invigorating influence on your facial muscles and skin, which elevates the "glowing" look and softens your skin's texture. Reversing the direction of gravity also helps lift and tighten unattractive sagging and drooping.

One more thing—always remember to empty your pockets ahead of time.

TAKE VITAMINS SPECIFICALLY FOR YOUR SKIN

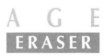

Please, don't *ever* believe those people who tell you that you can get all the vitamins and minerals you need from the food you eat. It's just not possible. Especially if you are attempting to be proactive and make improvements in specific aspects of your health and appearance such as your skin. You could never eat the quantity of food required daily to supply all the vitamins and minerals your body needs. The land we grow our food in is constantly being polluted, which compromises the quality of food produced, and so much of what the average person consumes has been processed to the point that the nutritional value is nil.

You *must* supplement your body's needs, and there are specific vitamins and minerals that contribute directly to your skin's well being. The important thing to remember, however, is to supplement your diet with a *balanced* intake of vitamins and minerals. Balanced supplementation is part of a complete nutrition program that contributes to a healthy body and healthy-looking skin.

Some specific vitamins and minerals that contribute to healthy skin include:

Vitamin A/Beta-Carotene

Vitamin A and beta-carotene are proven antioxidants. Vitamin A protects against the effects of radiation and pollution. It also helps maintain and repair skin and mucous membranes. Beta-carotene protects against ozone, smog, and toxic automobile emissions.

Vitamin B_2

Vitamin B_2 affects cell respiration and metabolism.

Vitamin B$_{12}$

Vitamin B$_{12}$ aids in cell formation and cellular longevity.

Vitamin C

Vitamin C offers some protection against radiation and is particularly necessary for tissue growth and repair.

Vitamin E

Vitamin E reduces the negative effects of LDL on cell membranes, and has been proven to reduce the long-term effects of aging.

Bioflavonoids

Bioflavonoids are not true vitamins in the strictest sense, but are sometimes referred to as Vitamin P. There are several different products and mixtures of bioflavonoids, including hesperidin, hesperetin, eriodictyol, quercetin, quercetrin, and rutin. The human body cannot produce bioflavonoids; they must be supplied in the diet. Bioflavonoids act synergistically with Vitamin C to protect and preserve the cell structure of capillary blood vessels.

Biotin

Biotin aids in cell growth and is needed for healthy hair and skin.

Folic Acid

Folic acid is a coenzyme in DNA synthesis and is important to healthy cell division and replication.

PABA

PABA is one of the basic constituents of folic acid. This antioxidant helps protect against sunburn and skin cancer. Supplementing with PABA may restore gray hair to its original color if stress or nutritional deficiency caused the graying.

Selenium

Recent studies of the mineral selenium show that increased intake may significantly reduce the risks of UV-induced skin cancer.

Niacin: Vitamin B$_3$

Taking niacin (Vitamin B$_3$) is important to the promotion of good blood circulation. Don't be frightened by the so-called niacin flush. Shortly after ingesting niacin, most people experience a tingling and flushed feeling. Some compare the sensation to a hot flash. I personally love the feeling. It tells me that my blood is getting to my skin's surface, promoting better circulation and a healthier appearance. Physicians have reported that some of their patients even use niacin to enhance sexual pleasure and regularly take their dose of niacin at bedtime. Whenever you take it, whether before a workout or before bedtime, know that the glow you feel is a desired reaction and your body is responding properly.

These are just some of the vitamins and minerals that contribute to your skin's well being and are essential to healthy, overall body functioning.

TAKE CARE OF YOUR SKIN— MORNING, NOON, AND NIGHT

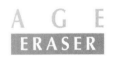

At a very young age I began buying skin-care products and treating my skin. I continue to do this faithfully. It is just as routine to me as brushing my teeth and shaving my face. One of the goals of my television show, and in this book, is to reach out to younger people. I want to share what is available to them right now, so they will not have to work as hard to push back the clock as those who may not have begun a lifestyle change until later in life.

I believe that my early use of "women's" cosmetics is an example of what I did to slow down the effects of aging. I want to specifically encourage young men to begin taking care of their skin early in life. Young girls start experimenting with cosmetics as soon as they see Mommy using them, and that behavior is reinforced their entire lifetime. It's acceptable and expected behavior for women. Some men still tend to limit their facial treatments to a quick slap of aftershave. Not so long ago it was considered less than manly to use creams and lotions. Lines and wrinkles were considered rugged and masculine.

While there is still a certain gender-related bias in society—men *do* get away with having more wrinkles as they age than the ladies do—the craggy-faced, wrinkle-browed Marlboro Man image is no longer in style. Fresh, healthy, and youthful-appearing skin is, and should be, the goal of everyone today.

My personal facial skin-care regime consists of three parts: morning treatments, an afternoon refresher, and evening treatments.

Every morning I exfoliate, cleanse, and moisturize my skin. As I said, I've experimented with literally hundreds of products. I strongly encourage everyone to take advantage of the free consultations that all major cosmetic companies offer. Only by experimentation will you find the products that best suit your particular skin.

Most cosmetic manufacturers market a three-part process that includes exfoliating, cleansing, and moisturizing as their basic skin-care system. This is where a professional consultation comes in handy. Learn about your skin so you know how to care for it. It is also important to reevaluate your skin-care regime any time you notice a major change. Weather, nutrition, water consumption, exercise, illness, prescription drugs—all of these can be a reason to evaluate and adjust your skin-care routine.

And guys, don't be afraid to sit up on that cosmetic-counter stool and let a consultant work on your face. Once you've tried it, you'll find that it's no different than going to the hairdresser or barbershop.

Though I personally consider shaving a necessary evil, it does provide two benefits to men that women do not share. First, it is an exfoliating process. The razor removes the top layer of dead skin cells as it removes the hair. Second, the very presence of hair follicles acts as a support system within the skin structure, keeping it thicker and stronger and less likely to sag. So there are some positives to that dreaded morning chore.

Exfoliating should be a regular part of daily skin care. There are a variety of interesting exfoliants, all in varying textures designed to work on specific body parts. A facial exfoliant is obviously much finer than one used on the feet. Use all exfoliants gently, but use them religiously. The living organism that is your skin needs to have all its dead cells removed regularly to look its best.

I cleanse my face with soap compounded especially for my skin type. There are hundreds of different cleansers—bars, liquids, creams—

all designed for various skin types. Find the one that is right for you and use it daily. It is critically important to start your day with clean skin, removing all traces of your nighttime treatments and the microscopic dust and dirt particles that have settled on your skin overnight.

Morning moisturizers should be light enough to not make your face shiny or oily looking, and for the ladies, should allow the easy application of your chosen makeup. Don't forget to gently moisturize the eye area. I always buy moisturizers specifically compounded for this sensitive area. Eye area moisturizers can be a little pricey but are a good investment because they last a long time and a little usually goes a long way.

And don't just moisturize your face. Your entire body should be treated after every shower or bath. Don't completely dry your body. Leave it damp and immediately apply moisturizing lotion over your damp skin. This added water will hydrate your skin even more intensely.

Morning treatments should always contain a high degree of UV protection. This is particularly important for men who (unless they are doing a television show) do not have the added protection of makeup. Protect your skin from harmful sun rays at all times. While I believe that a certain amount of exposure to the sun is acceptable and healthy looking, always remember that the sun is the number-one enemy of youthful skin, not to mention the major cause of skin cancer.

A couple of times a day I use a moisturizing mist. I keep a small spray bottle in my briefcase and in my car and gently spray my face and neck mid-morning and mid-afternoon. There are even fine mists that can be spritzed on over makeup.

In the evening I again exfoliate, cleanse, and moisturize. This is the time I use a heavier moisturizer. The old jokes about women going to bed with cold cream smeared all over their face could almost be told about me. I use the nighttime hours to deep moisturize and treat my skin. This is the time to fight the toll that the stresses of the day may have taken on your facial skin.

I frequently use a retinol treatment underneath my moisturizer. I have only used commercially available retinol treatments to date, which, with conscientious use, have produced a diminishing of fine lines. There are prescription formulas available that also produce very noticeable results on deeper lines and wrinkles. This, however, requires a physician's consultation and moves into the area of more invasive treatments.

The same people who ask me how I keep my skin looking so youthful, frequently have the same reaction when I tell them what I do—what

I've *always* done. They tell me they are too tired at night. They tell me they don't have enough time in the morning. Or, they say it's just too much trouble or too costly to do what I do.

Remember, we are talking about a lifestyle change here. A little effort will go a long way. You make time, you *schedule* time, for all the other things you consider important to take care of in your life. Isn't the person looking back at you in the mirror worth that kind of time commitment? Isn't it just as important to take care of you as it is to take care of your house, your car, your *lawn!* You maintain and treat all of these things. Aren't you more important than any of them? I think you are. And it's not being selfish to do this. Everyone benefits from a healthy and youthful lifestyle. The better you look and feel, the better you will treat everyone in your life. Looking your best is just one more part of a healthy lifestyle. It's time to make yourself a priority.

GET ENOUGH REST AND SLEEP

AGE ERASER

Every medical journal has recently written articles on sleep deprivation in the United States. We are a sleep-deprived nation and this is taking its toll on our health and our appearance. When a body is sleep deprived, it is not able to replenish and recover properly. Hormone functioning is disrupted. The whole magical biological rhythm of life is thrown off balance, and this is all reflected on our face. I can tell if I've had enough sleep (or too much sleep) just by looking in the mirror.

It's a very basic fact that to look your best you must be well rested. I believe we all have specific sleep needs that are personal to our own body chemistry. A healthy, well-cared-for body will determine its own needs. We just have to be cognizant of those needs, respect them, and be consistent in complying with them.

There are some very simple things you can do to get a good night's rest. Keep your bedroom for sex and sleep. Don't turn on the television, don't read, don't talk on the phone, don't work on your laptop computer, don't bring snacks to eat, and don't bring a briefcase full of work to bed with you. Avoid heavy meals, alcohol, and caffeine before bedtime. Either enjoy some intimate time with your partner and then relax and go to sleep, or just relax and go to sleep.

Sleeping on your back is best for your complexion, although some people find this difficult to do. Keep your hands below your heart. Hug a pillow if you tend to throw your arms up over your head when sleeping. This prevents undue stress on your heart. Use a night-light to help you see if you need to get up. Don't turn on a lamp, as this will disturb your brain's sleep pattern. If you simply cannot sleep, get up and leave the bedroom until you feel sleepy.

It's most important that you maintain a consistent sleep pattern, particularly on the weekend. Your body clock doesn't know Saturday morning from Tuesday morning. If you are tired during the day, take a 20- to 30-minute (not longer) nap. You'll awake fresh and ready to get on with your day, and isn't being able to take a short nap one of the nice things about a weekend anyway? When you are refreshed by plenty of undisturbed sleep, circles under your eyes disappear, wrinkles seem less severe, and the skin on your face seems to be more "alive" and vibrant.

BEFORE COSMETIC SURGERY, DO YOUR HOMEWORK

The age-erasing techniques that I've just explained are all relatively simple and not overly expensive. They can be done wherever your work or play takes you. They are the foundation of a good, sound, overall program to take care of your skin. Follow them and you will look and feel your best.

There are other skin-care options available that require a larger investment of time and money. These are the more invasive procedures known generally as plastic or cosmetic surgery. I personally feel that barring disease, accident, or injury, most cosmetic plastic surgery should not be done in your 20s, 30s, or even your early 40s.

Staying Forever Young does not mean eliminating every small wrinkle the minute it appears. It does not mean having perfect body proportions, or a movie star's complexion. If you take good care of your body, exercise, and eat properly you probably won't need cosmetic surgery for a good portion of your life. If you are a perfectionist and must have every body part in perfect proportion, you might want to take a second look at your priorities. A good plastic surgeon will help you assess and understand your underlying motivations and expectations and help you determine if they are realistic.

Which brings us to the most critical decision you will make if you decide to undergo one of these procedures: your choice of physician. Do your homework. Determine the credentials your potential plastic surgeon holds. Is he or she licensed? Is he board certified and, if so, for what specialties? What professional organizations does he belong to?

What hospitals grant him privileges? How many times has he performed the procedure you are considering? Ask for references from former patients. Ask to see before-and-after pictures of former patients. Again, a good plastic surgeon will happily answer all questions you may have, and will probably anticipate most of them.

All surgery carries with it certain inherent risks. The field of plastic and reconstructive surgery has come under criticism in the past, because not enough regulations governed who could perform certain procedures. When liposuction first gained popularity there were unscrupulous people, with minimal credentials, who tried to make fast money from performing the procedure. And, unfortunately, there were some patients looking for cut-rate deals. Some of these patients met with disastrous results. Some died. Plastic surgery, or, for that matter, any type of surgery, is not something that can or should be performed by just anyone. This is not the time to look for "the best deal."

Fortunately, there is now one organization whose endorsement of a physician indicates a certain level of expertise in the field. The American Society of Plastic and Reconstructive Surgeons states that their symbol by a physician's name designates "surgeons who are active members of the American Society of Plastic and Reconstructive Surgeons. They are certified in the specialty of plastic surgery by the American Board of Plastic Surgery and are dedicated to the highest standards of patient welfare and surgical excellence."

Once you feel comfortable with your choice of physician, you must listen to what he or she tells you and be honest about your expectations. A good plastic surgeon will assess your overall health and discuss your specific goals in detail. He will not hesitate to decline to perform a procedure if he feels your expectations are unrealistic. You should be frank in discussing everything with your physician. He or she should be equally frank with you, describing alternatives and the risks and limitations of each.

The spectrum of cosmetic surgery available today includes so many procedures that to properly describe them all would take several books on that subject alone. Some of the less invasive procedures include: CO_2 laser treatment, erbium laser treatment, spider vein removal laser treatment, power peels, micro-dermabrasion, laser resurfacing, phenol and TCA (trichloroacetic acid) peels, and botox injections.

Cosmetic surgery of the head and neck includes procedures such as rhinoplasty (nose job), rhytidectomy (face-lift), blepharoplasty (eyelids), otoplasty (ear reshaping), facial implants (forehead, cheeks, chin, lips, brows, jaw), chemical peels, dermabrasion, forehead and brow lifts, facial and neck liposuction, and hair replacement surgery.

Other procedures include breast augmentation (implants), buttock augmentation (implants), breast reduction, breast reconstruction, breast lift, liposuction of the stomach, thighs, buttocks, back, and arms, and abdominoplasty (tummy tuck).

If you have the financial resources, and the time needed for recovery, there is a procedure for just about every fault you can find with your body. Just be judicious in your choice of physician and realistic in your expectations of outcome.

MAKE SKIN CARE A PRIORITY

Your skin is the cover, the outer garment of your body. You wouldn't expose the rest of your body by going out into subzero temperatures without the protection of a warm coat or jacket. You wouldn't go out into the heat of the desert sun naked. Don't expose your face to temperature extremes without protection either. Use your cleansers, moisturizers, sunscreens, and lotions. And if you take nothing else from my suggestions in this chapter, drink lots of water—preferably distilled—every day. None of my age-erasing tips for the skin will do more for you as quickly as drinking at least half of your body weight in ounces of water every day.

Your skin requires more time and attention because it is the largest organ of your body. It is the shield between your body and the billions of foreign substances out in the atmosphere waiting to attack you. It's what others see first, before they have time to get to know you personally. Make proper skin care a priority in your age-erasing lifestyle change.

six

bone up with bill: strong, healthy bones for life

A s you get older, a healthy skeletal structure is fundamental to the fullness of your life. You should be able to stand up straight no matter what your age. You should be able to play tennis, climb a mountain, and even jump on a trampoline your entire life. Decide today that you're *not* going to end up all hunched over and so brittle that you can't even sit up straight and watch your favorite television program (which I hope is Bill Frank's *Forever Young*!). Make the commitment to change the behavioral patterns that are allowing your bones to grow thin and turn brittle.

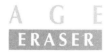

UNDERSTAND THAT NEW BONE *CAN* BE BUILT

How much bone mass have you lost in the last 10 to 20 years? That depends on your body chemistry, your diet, and your level and type of physical activity. Most people now believe that you can stop bone loss if you know how. The big misconception is that once it's gone, you can't build it back. Not true!

I've seen numerous medical studies that verify your body's ability to increase bone density, all the way up into your 90s. That is very good news; especially considering the prevalence and devastation of osteoporosis.

Consider the following: Research has shown that, on average, an adult loses 1 percent of bone mass per year. Among women, bone loss increases tenfold after menopause. Many women have lost 30 percent of their bone mass by their 60th birthday. One-fifth of all women have had skeletal fractures by age 70.

As far as I'm concerned, this is about 30 to 40 years too early to have your capacity for vibrant, active living destroyed by chronic bone loss. *As bad as the problem is, incredibly, this is an epidemic that can be wiped out with some very basic and uncomplicated steps.*

Tufts University conducted research in which they asked elderly patients, all of them over 75 years of age, to do simple weight-bearing exercises such as leg extensions and leg curls for four weeks. Tufts was actually testing the ability of seniors to increase muscular strength and size. The oldest patient was 96 years old. Could this person possibly increase strength at this age? And if he increased strength, is it even remotely possible that he could increase muscle density or build new muscle tissue?

Lo and behold, the answer was yes, yes, and yes! Not only did many of the subjects experience 100 percent strength increases; they also increased muscle density by up to 90 percent. And yes, several people in that test were able to build additional muscle tissue, including the 96-year-old man.

This was excellent news. But what came next is the truly amazing part of this story. They discovered something that they weren't even studying. In running the MRIs and other clinical tests, they had recorded the subjects' bone density levels prior to the test. When they tested the new muscle density levels, almost incidentally, they also remeasured the subjects' bone density levels. The results were remarkable: *In 93 percent of these patients, their bone density also increased.*

Now, if this can happen to someone who is in their 80s or 90s, just imagine what it could do for you in your 20s, 30s, 40s, 50s, or wherever you may be along this walk of life. Why not spend the next 10 years strengthening your skeletal structure instead of standing by and watching it wither and wilt away?

I don't like hearing people explaining the onset of frailty with the excuse, "Well, you know, after all, I'm 50 years old. I've been here a half century." I tell them, "I don't care how long you have been on this earth when it comes to staying strong." How long has the Mississippi River been here and it's still raging? How long has the Pacific Ocean been here and it's still pounding the sandy beaches of the coast? I don't want to hear people say how long they've been here. I want them looking forward to just how long they are going to remain healthy.

GET A BONE DENSITY TEST

First, you want to find out exactly how your skeletal structure is doing. This is an excellent biomarker of your body's real physiological age—few things are more basic to your overall health and well-being than your bones. You'll find out how aggressive your intervention needs to be—or if you just need to focus on prevention.

Ask your physician to advise you of a hospital or clinic near you that can perform this simple but eye-opening test. Once you know how dense your bones are at this stage of your life, you can keep track of your progress as you institute a bone-strengthening program. Once you know your level, you can take control and manage your bone density, just like other aspects of your health. Anything that *can* be measured *should* be measured, so you can strive to keep it moving in the right direction. I assure you, you *will* be able to add bone mass each year, instead of losing it.

LOAD-BEARING EXERCISE: THE MORE INTENSE THE BETTER

In a famous scientific essay called "Disuse and Aging," Dr. Walter M. Bortz came to the conclusion that "at least a portion of the changes that are commonly attributed to aging are, in reality, caused by immobility. As such, they're subject to correction by mobility—meaning activity and exercise."

This couldn't be more true of the debilitating disease most frequently attributed to old age: osteoporosis. In simple terms, you need to press and pull and tug on your bones with your muscles. Challenge them constantly and with intensity. Like most organs in your body, they will respond when they are needed. They will get stronger and thicker. Numerous medical studies document this fact.

Many people think of bones as hard, static, inanimate structures, just like the skeletons hanging in the doctor's office. But in reality, bone is active, living tissue—changing all the time and reacting to internal and external stimuli that we provide. When you understand this, you can get a picture of how you can influence the health of your bones through exercise and nutrition.

I perform load-bearing exercises three or four times a week, especially those exercises that affect my hips, my thighs, my calves, and my ankles—the foundation of my body that supports every move. Whether I am walking or running, on a flat surface or up a set of stairs, it really doesn't matter. These are the wheels and the tires of my body. If *they* don't go, *I* don't go. So as a result, I need to make sure that three to four times a week they are getting demanding, physical exercise.

By *demanding*, I simply mean that they are being put to unusual tests that they are not put to during normal activities like walking around or going up a flight of stairs. It requires load-bearing exercises to really challenge and change your bones.

These should be intense load-bearing exercises. Generally, 70–80 percent of the maximum weight you can lift is what would be considered high intensity for you.

The biomechanics that explain how exercise builds bone density start with your neurotransmission system. It goes back to our fright-flight reaction. If we are challenged, there are nerve centers in the brain that direct endorphins to go out and prepare us for danger. Our body reacts to how much we have to handle. It appears that our bones work in exactly the same way. Once they get comfortable, they get stagnant. They become very accustomed to our normal activity level. What was once difficult for us becomes easy. You must challenge your bones, as well as your muscles, ligaments, and tendons to do additional work. This will enable them to get bigger and to get stronger.

The fact that something is pushing against the bone, and the bone is pushing back at it, forces this bone to say, "Hey, I have to work harder. I have to be stronger to do this or I'm going to break or buckle." As a result, the body, in all of its infinite wisdom, makes the bone stronger and increases its density, allowing it to push whatever weight it eventually decide it wants to push.

Now many of you, especially women, are going to say, "Bill, I'm 50 years old. I've never touched a weight in my life. That's just not me."

Well I'm here to say, it *can* be you. A few years ago I began to train a woman who was in her mid-50s and decided she was going to do a reversal. This was a woman who walked like an old woman—shuffling along, very weak and frail. Prior to starting to train, she had allowed herself to get 70 pounds overweight. She had this beautiful face, was intelligent, bright, and loved by many. But she had a growing disdain for herself and this seemed to affect her relationship with others.

One of the things I noted in the training process, aside from the fact that she developed a better personality and lost a good 60 pounds, was how much stronger she actually became each week. Remember that this was not a 25- or 35-year-old woman. This woman was 50-plus, perhaps about the same age as you.

As hard as it may be to believe, in the beginning it was difficult for her to lie on a leg-press machine and press more than 50–75 pounds, which at that time was probably close to one-third of her body weight. Within a year, this lady was leg pressing over 400 pounds. Within a year and a half, she was leg pressing over 500 pounds.

This was a woman who decided that she wanted to do something about it. And now this woman has great strength, walks straight up, and has no problems with broken or brittle bones. Her bone density tests have improved in each of the four tests she has taken in the past eighteen months. If you met this woman, you would see a healthy, energetic, attractive, trim person. You would never know how much weight she lifts or how much bone density she has added. But *she* knows, and it has made her a very happy person.

AGE
ERASER

EXERCISES THAT STIMULATE HEALTHY HORMONES

Now, for you really motivated students, I'm going to take you to the next level of bone density builders. There are some exercises that have been shown to increase the release of your body's hGH or human growth hormones. As we have explained in this book, one of the primary causes of many aging symptoms is the steady decline in your body's release of hGH as you age.

It is widely accepted among physicians that certain intense exercises will naturally stimulate hormonal release. Seems like a simple solution to a lot of aging problems, doesn't it? The problem is that millions of baby boomers never, ever, partake in intense exercise. Those of you who decide to start will be rewarded with stronger bones and a host of other benefits that will keep your body performing at younger levels.

EXERCISES THAT INCREASE HORMONE LEVELS

There are five exercises that tests have shown will increase hormone levels, especially hGH, in your body. These are all "heavy" exercises. But remember, "heavy" is relative. If it is heavy for you, then you are using enough to stimulate the results we are seeking. You should use enough weight with each exercise that you have to struggle to do four or five repetitions. Demonstrations of all five exercises begin on page 100.

Warning: You will be tired when you are done, because you will be struggling with even five repetitions. But it will be well worth the effort, because test after test proves that these exercises increase the release of hGH in your body, which supports muscle density, bone density, increased circulation, and more effective and efficient use of oxygen. If you had the time, you could have your blood work done before and after your workout, and be able to read the healthy difference right there in black and white.

Again, I'm not trying to turn you into a weight lifter like me. But the benefits to your body and your overall health are indisputable. And when you leave the gym, your sense of vitality, confidence, and overall well-being are an instant reward.

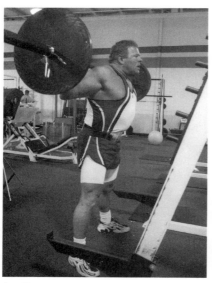 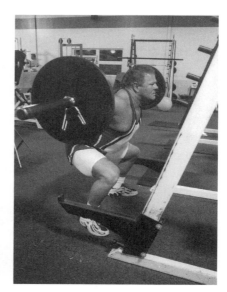

Leg Squats

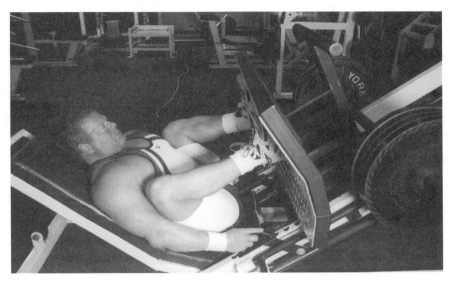

Leg Press

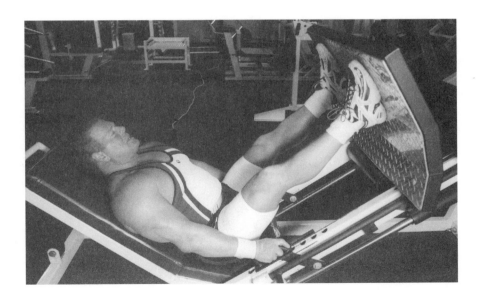

➤ HORMONE-LEVEL EXERCISES (CONTINUED)

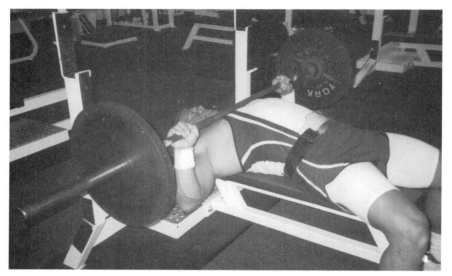

Bench Press

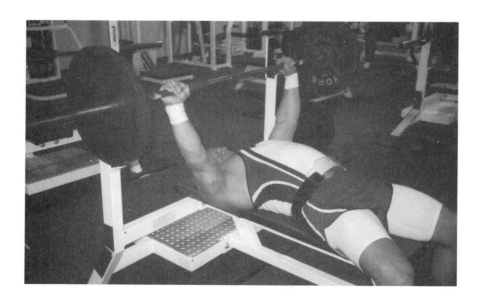

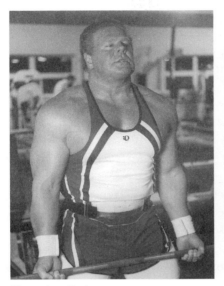 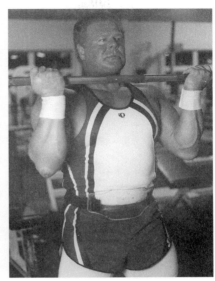

Heavy Arm Curls

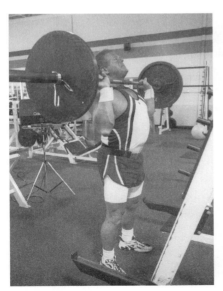 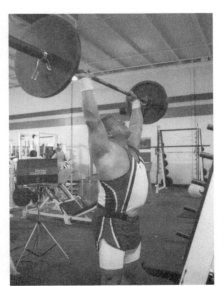

Military Press

EXERCISES FOR THE SPINE

Many scientists believe that the spine is the fastest aging part of the body. This is because the neurotransmission activity is so great. The spine is where everything comes and goes. It is the center of the parasympathetic and the sympathetic nervous system. It is the home of the autonomic nervous system. Of course, it is the structural center and the nerve center that supports the entire body and all of the signals to the body coming from the brain.

I want you to add a few spine exercises to keep this critical part of your body vibrant. I do an exercise called "good mornings." I put an Olympic-style barbell using light to moderate weight on my shoulders with my legs slightly flexed but locked. Then I bend over with that weight until I am at a 90-degree angle from the floor. Then I come back up. This is a great strengthener of the low spine and it's also a stretcher of the spine. See the spine exercises on pages 105–106.

Hyper-extension exercises are great for the spine. Flexibility is also one of the major things you want to consider for a healthier spine. One reason I am so big on leg and hip exercises is that a strong lower body helps cushion your spine. However, if you are doing leg presses, squats, or things that strengthen the hips and the legs, then you are doing exercises that in some way compact the spine, so you need to stretch your spine out too. You need to do exercises like pull-ups, because you are pulling the other way as you stretch the spine out. Also add in some pull-downs on a lat machine—and make use of the long-pull machine for your lower and internal back to stretch and thicken the spine out as far as you can.

Remember, gravity is pulling your spine down for all the hours that you are upright and not lying on your back, so you want to do all that you can to reverse the effects of gravity and to build strength the other way. This will provide the best possible benefit of muscle density and bone density for the overall body.

The leg exercises that I outlined earlier are also important to a healthy spine. I have told professional athletes for years: "Your careers are as long as your legs are strong."

Strong legs with firm, flexible muscles protect your back, serving as a shock absorber during all of the physical activities in your life. They are the foundation of the body and they support your spine. So start your workouts there, then work yourself up and make sure that your back and spine are also flexible and strong.

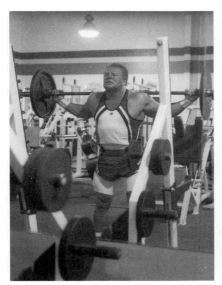 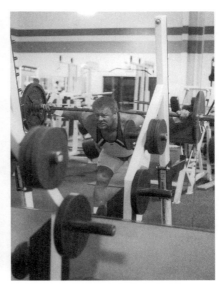

Good Mornings

➤ **SPINE EXERCISES (CONTINUED)**

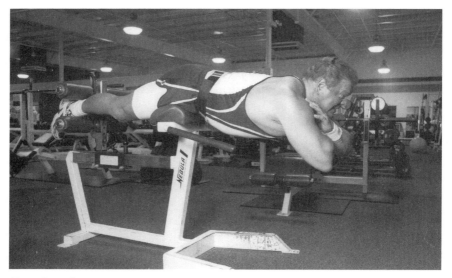

Hyper-Extensions

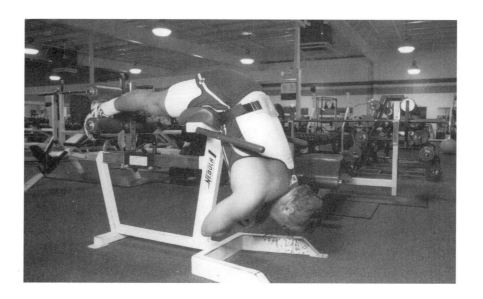

A RADICAL IDEA: DRINK MILK

Of all my recommendations, ironically, this is probably the one that some people will resist the most. Think of it. When is the last time you saw an adult order a glass of milk in a restaurant? Have you ever seen this? Does it seem possible that this bizarre milk aversion among adults, especially among women, could be related to the prevalence of the osteoporosis epidemic in America?

Remember breakfast cereal? It's the stuff in a bowl you used to eat in the mornings when you were a child. It's fast, tastes good, and is a great way to get milk in your system. I eat a bowl of Cheerios or Total every day, which gives me lots of essential vitamins and minerals. And it gives me milk. You ought to try this *revolutionary* combination.

I believe that we ought to drink milk as long as we are alive. When I was a boy, I drank fresh cow's milk, right from the farm. We didn't have a lot of broken bones when we were kids because everybody drank milk from my Uncle John's farm. We thought, "this is cool." And we had real whole milk. It was so good for us, because it had an incredible amount of protein, calcium, phosphorus, and Vitamin D.

As time went on, doctors began to tell us that we didn't need milk beyond the nurturing ages. I often ask myself out of common sense, "why have we diminished the value of milk in our minds?" Most human beings, at somewhere between 2 and 3 years of age, have reached one-half the height that they are going to be as an adult.

Hard to believe, but think about it. If a little boy reaches 3 feet tall by the time he's 3 years old, sure enough, you see him as a man and there he is, about 6 feet or 6-feet-1. You see somebody who is about 2-feet-5 or 2-feet-6 at age 3, and chances are, he's going be 5-feet-2 or 5-feet-6 when he's fully grown. And yet, remember, during those first years, what was the staple that baby lived on and survived on—was it not milk? Just think how much we rely on milk for the early development of our brain, our heart, our kidneys, our spleen, and the rest of our internal organs.

Milk plays a vital role early, and yet as we grow and put our body under enormous stress, both physical and mental, somehow someone would like to convince us that we no longer need milk. Isn't this a shame?

Yes, milk has calories and some fat, and a few people are lactose intolerant. But you have such easy options, especially with the availability of low-fat and nonfat milk, as well as goat's milk and lactose-free milk. Milk is a great nutritional bargain with very few negative effects.

AGE ERASER

BONE-BUILDING FOODS AND SUPPLEMENTS

Beyond milk, are you getting enough foods that are rich in calcium, phosphorus, potassium, and magnesium? Are you taking in ample levels of Vitamin D? Following are the Forever Young bone builders—foods that will keep your skeletal structure young and strong. You will also find the recommended levels of each nutrient I advise for optimum bone health.

Calcium

Bones are made of collagen and calcium phosphate. Over 80 percent of us have diets that are calcium deficient. So this is the most critical place to start. In addition to two glasses of milk per day, I recommend foods like yogurt (452 mg of calcium per serving), cheese (355 mg), tofu (435 mg), sardines (272 mg), salmon (242 mg), almonds (94 mg), spinach (122 mg), watermelon (617 mg), kale (90 mg), broccoli (89 mg), okra (88 mg), and beets (82 mg). Recommended level: The National Institutes of Health recommends 1000 mg of calcium per day for premenopausal women, 1200 mg per day for pregnant women, and 1500 per day for postmenopausal women and for men over 65. I recommend 1500 mg a day for everyone.

I encourage you to eat a calcium-rich diet, but you should come to grips with the fact that it is highly unlikely that you are getting what you need in food alone. Schedules are too demanding to get enough of the right foods, and the foods that you do eat are often too depleted of nutrients. Also, lots of things we consume deplete our calcium levels, which makes supplementation even more critical. The most common offenders are salt, caffeine, fat, alcohol, and tobacco.

So find yourself a high-quality supplement—the most natural and complete you can find. Many calcium supplements also include magnesium and phosphorus, two of the other nutrients that promote healthy bones. I would take half of the supplements with breakfast, and half before bed.

Vitamin C

In addition to being a powerful antioxidant, high doses of Vitamin C increase the production of collagen and increase the repair and replacement of all connective tissues, including bone tissue. This is why I feel so strongly about drinking two glasses of orange juice every day. There is no better natural source of Vitamin C. I like to put milk on my cereal, and accompany it with a large glass of orange juice. Recommended level: 1000–3000 mg daily for maximum bone repair.

Folic Acid

As I have stated in another chapter, folic acid (or folates) helps prevent the buildup of homocysteine, which not only leads to heart disease, but is also a risk factor for osteoporosis. This is another reason to drink orange juice every day and to make certain you eat your cruciferous vegetables, such as broccoli and brussels sprouts.

Zinc

Zinc is necessary in cell growth and protein synthesis, and is involved in the function of the endocrine glands—adrenal, prostate, pancreas, etc. Zinc binds to protein and bone in the body. It aids wound healing and is an anti-inflammatory that helps treat arthritis and other autoimmune diseases. Common sources in foods are meat, shellfish, liver, eggs, poultry, black-eyed peas, soybeans, and peanuts. Recommended level: 50 mg daily.

Magnesium

Magnesium is required in a comparatively large quantity—magnesium deficiency is very common in America today. As much as 50 percent of all the magnesium in the body is found in the structure of the bones, so a deficiency will certainly influence the health of your skeletal structure. In studies in which magnesium was added to estrogen replacement therapy in postmenopausal women, bone density levels increased 11 percent over a nine-month period, compared to 0.7 percent in women taking the estrogen alone. It is found in foods such as soybeans, dried peas, lentils, whole grains, shellfish, nuts, and kelp. Recommended level: 400 mg daily.

Manganese

Manganese is a catalyst for enzyme systems. Henry Shroder, M.D., and George Cotzias, M.D., leaders in the field of trace minerals, found manganese to be essential for bone and tendon metabolism. It is plentiful in bran, nuts, and whole-grain cereals. As with magnesium, the highest concentrations in the human body is found in the bones and in various endocrine glands. Recommended level: 20 mg daily.

Vitamin D

Vitamin D is an important partner to calcium as it aids in absorption. Vitamin D strengthens bones, prevents joint deterioration, and may help offset the onset and aging effects of arthritis. Only a few foods naturally contain Vitamin D: tuna, salmon, sardines, oysters. We need 10–20 minutes of sunlight exposure each day to trigger the chemical reaction that creates usable Vitamin D. Recommended level: 600 IU daily.

Phosphorus

People suffering from a deficiency in phosphorus are rare. The more likely scenario is an excess of phosphorus, usually from consuming too much junk food. Phosphorus is required, in balance with magnesium and calcium, for bone, cell, and tooth formation, kidney function, and proper heart muscle contraction. Asparagus, bran, corn, dairy foods, eggs, fish, nuts, seeds, meats, poultry, and salmon all contain fair amounts of phosphorus. Excessive amounts of phosphorus will inhibit calcium uptake.

Boron

Boron is also needed for calcium uptake, but only in trace amounts. As with phosphorus, the normal person is not usually deficient in boron. However, because absorption of calcium becomes more difficult as we age, we can benefit from increased boron intake in our middle years. Supplementing with 3 mg of boron has proven beneficial to men and women over 40. Boron is found naturally in grains, fruits, nuts, and vegetables. Recommended dosage: not more than 3 mg daily.

BO KNOWS THE VALUE OF STRONG BONES, YOU SHOULD TOO

I take care of my bones because I don't want to be bent over or lose my stride when I'm walking. I don't want to shuffle. I want to be able to pick my feet up and down. I want to be able to bend my knees. I want my hips to rotate. I want my skeletal structure to remain in this state throughout my life.

Look at the great, great athlete Bo Jackson. He was the "Just Do It" man for Nike. You could not turn on the TV without seeing commercials featuring Bo Jackson's remarkable multi-sport athletic feats. Bo Jackson can't buy a commercial today. Why? Because he suffered a major injury that required a hip replacement and severely limited his mobility and ability. His is a graphic example of what happens to someone who can't perform in a society that puts such a high value on performance.

Now this artificial hip will allow him to move around and live a fairly normal life. But what is a normal life? It's certainly not normal for Bo Jackson, who could run a 100-meter dash in 9.9 seconds and could do things that few other men could. But once he had that hip injury it all changed. Do you think Bo thought about the importance of healthy bone mass before his debilitating problem?

It's the same with millions of people today. We just don't think about these bones of ours that are so critical to the future quality of our lives. You can sneak by without any thought in your 20s, 30s, and 40s. But sooner or later it's going to catch up with you, and it's going to be a hard landing.

In the most severe cases, people fall down, break a hip, and some of them actually die because their whole skeletal structure has atrophied. Others end up slowed down, hunched over, immobile, and incapable of swinging a driver or smashing a forehand.

That's not going to happen to me. And I certainly don't want it to happen to you. When I'm 75 or 80, I'm going to walk tall, with a strong gait and my head high. Are you going to join me?

seven
how to keep your memory and maintain a healthy brain

WITH DR. CASS TERRY

Dr. Cass Terry is one of the more prominent physicians and a leading expert in the field of age management. This not only encompasses the study of the mind, the brain, and memory system that he writes about in this chapter, but also includes the field of endocrinology and hormone replacement therapy. Dr. Terry's medical opinions and views are included in this chapter and nowhere else in this book. Although Dr. Terry endorses the principles described throughout this book, he does not endorse the hormone replacement therapy or any clinic referenced in the chapter on hormone replacement therapy.

f, throughout the history of time, mankind has believed that the human body is a difficult and complex structure to understand, then certainly he has been mystified and overwhelmed with the complexities of the human brain. From the first time that we open our eyes or babble our first *mama* or *dada*, flex a muscle, or make use of any one of the senses available to us, our brain is in control. It's no wonder then that the most devastating and frightening experience we ever face is when our brain begins to lose some of its capacity to function at optimum levels.

This was brought home to me with a vengeance when our family doctor said to me, "Bill, your mother has Alzheimer's disease." At that time I remember thinking that I possessed some understanding of the disease. I guess what I really thought was that Alzheimer's disease was just another word for dementia, and that my mother was simply entering the early stages of senility. Because of this terrible disease, my mother's body was in its seventh decade, but her mind was somewhere back remembering experiences from her late teens. As time passed, I realized that the person I knew and loved, and who physically appeared to be a completely healthy woman, only sometimes recognized my face as someone she ought to know. And even then she wasn't sure whether I was her son, her father, or a young man she wanted to flirt with. If it weren't so horrible, it might have been cute or funny.

Because of this personal experience, I wanted the information in this chapter on the healthy brain to come from one of the foremost authorities I could possibly find. Recently, Dr. L. Cass Terry, M.D., Ph.D., Pharm.D., joined my company as medical director and director of research and development. Dr. Terry was the chairman of neurology and professor of physiology and endocrinology at a leading midwestern medical college. He is one of the world's leading experts on aging and the brain. He has directed several landmark age-prevention studies and has published over 130 papers, book chapters, and abstracts in the field. I am very proud and grateful that Dr. Terry agreed to provide me with the latest scientific breakthroughs in the vital area of memory retention and age-management techniques for the brain. Like any good tour guide I want you to receive the highest quality information—information that may prevent you or someone you love from experiencing firsthand, as I have with my mother, the debilitating and devastating effects of brain failure. Therefore, all of the credit for the information I am about to share with you goes to Dr. Cass Terry. In this chapter he is the expert; I am merely the messenger!

We don't yet have the ability to reverse the aging of our brain, but that doesn't mean we can't slow down the aging process to the best of our capability. There is a big difference between aging and becoming old! As stated by David Mahoney and Richard Restak, becoming old means:

➤ accepting the notion that it's too late to change
➤ believing that life doesn't matter anymore
➤ failing to set goals and commitments
➤ losing interest in life
➤ losing a sense of surprise and giving in to boredom

It is not inevitable that you will become biologically old. There are several measures you can take to prevent or slow down the aging of your brain. The first and foremost concept to grasp is that prevention is of the utmost importance. The longer we wait to intervene, the more function we will lose, and it may be irreversible if left unattended for too long. By the time someone reaches the level of diagnosable Alzheimer's disease (AD), there is very little that can be done to restore normal brain function. Another thing—you must realize that there are no prescription drugs approved to treat early-onset memory loss, because the Federal Drug Administration (FDA) doesn't recognize it as a disease, and pharmaceutical companies can't seek FDA approval of a drug unless it is for treatment of a specific disease.

There are a large number of people in their sixth decade of life who begin to notice difficulties with their memories. Symptoms might include inability to recall or identify faces and names, telephone numbers, pager numbers, etc. This difficulty tends to increase with time and interfere with work and social interactions. The condition has been called age-associated memory impairment (AAMI) or it is sometimes referred to as ARMI (age-related memory impairment). More recently, a condition called mild cognitive impairment (MCI) was described. It is basically a short-term memory problem without any other cognitive loss. MCI is believed to be the forerunner to Alzheimer's disease, because a large percentage of individuals with MCI will develop AD within three years.

Developing a dysfunctional brain is one of our greatest fears as we age. In focus groups, comprised of people in their sixth decade or older, the majority state that what they fear most, above all else as they age, is loss of their memory and cognitive skills. In general, most people feel they would be better off if they could improve their memory even a little bit.

THE BRAIN: SIMPLE CONCEPTS ABOUT THE MOST COMPLICATED ORGAN IN OUR BODY

Our brains are unlike any of our other organs, because each tiny region has a very specialized function that is not duplicated anywhere else. So if we sustain an injury to even a very small area of our brain, we can end up with some deficits that severely compromise our ability to function. Even with all of our high-tech supercomputers, the brain is still the most efficient and complicated computer. It has yet to be duplicated and it sure can't be transplanted! So we must do everything possible to preserve it.

In order to do that, we have to understand how the brain and nerve cells function. An individual brain cell is called a *neuron*. It has a body that receives information from other neurons and, in turn, produces a response that is sent out to other nerve cells or muscles to generate a thought, movement, vision, smell, taste, tears, or perspiration, etc. Neurons receive information through thousands of little processes called *dendrites*, which are best visualized as heavily branched bushes with the roots attached to the cell body.

Information is sent out by a long extension of the cell called the *axon*. Each nerve cell has only one axon sheathed by a thin coating called *myelin*. This is best visualized as a copper wire with insulation wrapped around it. Myelin is essential for most nerve cells to conduct electricity normally, otherwise the electricity will ground out. The axon then makes contact with another cell of one type or another through a junction box called a *synapse*. It communicates with the next cell down the line by releasing a chemical messenger into the synapse that, in turn, is taken up and activates that cell. The chemical messengers are called *neurotransmitters*. One nerve cell can be connected to thousands of other nerve cells through the dendrites.

Your brain has certain basic needs that must be met in order for it to function properly: First, it needs fuel, and that fuel is glucose. The brain cannot survive long without glucose. Hypoglycemia (low blood sugar) can cause significant brain damage after only a short period of time.

Second, your brain needs oxygen to burn the fuel, which is carried to it through the cerebral blood vessels: the carotid and vertebral arteries. So, your heart must pump blood to the brain and your arteries must be open to allow it to reach the brain. If either of these systems malfunctions, your brain can be permanently damaged in a relatively short period of time (five minutes).

Third, your brain needs amino acids, minerals, electrolytes, vitamins, hormones, and fatty acids to manufacture neurotransmitters, stabilize electrical potentials, maintain metabolic functions, preserve myelin, and strengthen cell walls. Many, if not most, of these brain nutrients decline as we age and, therefore, require supplementation.

In order to prevent memory and cognitive loss, we must first know what causes it. There are many theories, the most popular of which has to do with oxidative damage to cells and cell membranes. In other words, oxidation of fatty acids in nerve cell walls and damage to the mitochondria (the power house of the cell) tends to cause accumulation of damaged materials, loss of dendrites, sick and dying cells, and ultimately cell death. This could manifest as Alzheimer's or Parkinson's disease, depending on the regions most damaged. Other theories about the cause of memory loss involve programmed cell death, and the formation of neurotoxins from ingested materials in food, water, and the atmosphere. Deficiencies of one or more brain nutrients can also result in memory loss and eventual cell death, if not recognized and treated.

Arteriosclerosis and high blood pressure can also cause cumulative brain damage that will eventually manifest itself as a memory loss. Accumulation of tiny small infarcts (strokes) will eventually result in decreased memory and cognitive function.

Lifestyle and the Healthy Brain

Another completely different school of thought is that memory loss and Alzheimer's disease are due to lifestyle. Dharma Singh Khalsa, M.D., in his book *Brain Longevity*, says that chronic stress causes continued excessive concentrations of hydrocortisone, which, in turn, is toxic to brain cells. He and others believe that reducing your stress and maintaining a balanced and happy spirit are critical to the preservation of a well-functioning mind (See Chapter Thirteen).

But here is what is important: *Cognitive losses are not an inevitable outcome of aging. Crystallized intelligence*, such as vocabulary and general information, increases with age. On the other hand, *fluid intelligence*, including perceptual speed and information-processing speed and memory span, in general, declines with age. *Explicit memory*, the intention to remember, and the subsequent ability to recall a specific name, number, or location on demand, declines with age. However, there is a tremendous variation in the age that most people begin to experience a decline in any specific cognitive ability.

In order to begin our Forever Young program to improve brain function and prevent memory loss, we have to be able assess and follow our functioning over time. As the saying goes, "You can't manage it if you can't measure it."

Your memory and other cognitive skills can be tested in several different ways. The most extensive method is neuropsychological testing, which takes from three to six hours and is relatively expensive. The other extreme is the seven-minute screen or the MMSE (mini–mental status exam). The problem with the MMSE is that it is not very sensitive and does not pick up early loss of function, when we can do the most to prevent it.

Recently, a new device has been developed that allows individuals and/or their caregivers to easily gain access to the cognitive skills that tend to decline with age. It is part of the BrainCare Network and it can be tried without cost on their web site, which is www.brain.com. The primary testing device is called Thinkfast. It has several tests that assess the following:

- reaction time
- perceptual reflexes (visual acuity, alertness, and reaction speed)
- short-term memory
- working memory speed (your brain's speed of memory access)
- working memory capacity (your short-term "working" memory)
- visual-spatial reflexes (your brain's data-processing speed)
- delayed memory (your ability to keep track of several things at the same time)
- immediate memory (the speed with which you can remember something you've just seen)

These tests can be taken at any time in your home with your personal computer. They allow you to compare your performances over time and can be downloaded to a site that can be accessed by a caregiver. Using this device, whatever age-eraser program you decide upon can be tested and followed over time for its efficacy.

Using these tests over several weeks can improve your mental performance and keep your skills in maximum shape—the same thing you do for your body with aerobic and resistance training. The tests can also enhance your athletic performance and improve your competitive edge.

How Can We Maximize Brain Fitness?

Well, now that we know how the brain works, what happens to it with age, and how to measure its function, we can look at programs designed to maximize brain fitness. To keep it simple, we have to make sure our brain gets adequate glucose, maximum blood supply, all the substances necessary to maximize neurotransmitter function, vitamins, minerals, antioxidants for protection from neurotoxins, and certain hormones. Other agents called *nootropics* are believed to enhance cognitive function. Exactly how they work in the body is not known with certainty, but many have had documented success.

One of the wonderful things happening in the world of wellness today is that a growing number of caring and educated physicians have become acutely aware of the fact that there are nutrients available, outside of the prescription drug arena, that can be extremely valuable to anyone pursuing optimal wellness in their efforts to remain Forever

Young. As a result, these physicians have become strong advocates of recommending certain vitamins and minerals along with antioxidants to enhance your health and wellness.

On the following pages you will find charts with information about some very essential vitamins and nutrients that are vital to a healthy brain, as well as a suggested daily dose. Begin to include these recommendations in your daily life and you'll enjoy a measurable increase in the health of your brain. And remember, it's extremely important to be able to measure your progress after two or three months of a particular supplement, hormone, or nootropic. We suggest you use the brain.com system mentioned earlier in this chapter to keep an accurate record of your mental acuity before and after implementing our suggestions for a healthy brain.

As a final comment, I encourage you to read *every day*. Read books about anything and everything that interests you. Read anything that you find educational, stimulating, and thought-provoking. Put jigsaw puzzles together. Work difficult math problems and challenging crossword puzzles. And above all, read inspiring works that motivate you.

Remember, your brain, just like the muscle in your legs and arms, is stimulated and strengthened through controlled use and exercise. If it receives the same care and treatment as those muscles, it's possible to keep your brain, along with the rest of your body, Forever Young!

SUPPLEMENTS FOR BRAIN HEALTH

SUPPLEMENTS RECOMMENDED FOR A HEALTHY BRAIN

SUPPLEMENT	FUNCTION	DAILY DOSE
Vitamin B Complex (B_1, B_3, B_5, B_6, B_{12})	Promotes healthy nervous system and maximum mental performance.	1000 mg twice daily
Vitamin C	Prevents oxidative damage to nerve cells; vital to neurotransmitter production.	Highly variable; 1–4 g divided into 3–4 doses
Vitamin E	Prevents heart and brain deterioration; reduces oxidative stress; slows progression of AD.	No more than 800–1000 IU daily

NOOTROPICS FOR A HEALTHY BRAIN

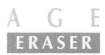

Nootropics are believed to improve learning, memory consolidation, and memory retrieval, without side effects. There are several of these agents; some of their mechanisms of action are not known with certainty, but many have had documented success.

NOOTROPIC	FUNCTION	DAILY DOSE
Pyroglutamic acid	Improves verbal memory after 60 days' use; stimulates cognitive function; fights anxiety. More effective when paired with CDP-choline.	500 mg 3 times a day
CDP-choline	Helps brain manufacture neuro-transmitters; retards progression of AD; increases blood circulation and oxygen utilization in brain; alleviates depression; improves learning ability and memory.	Under physician's care: 250 mg 2 times a day for 30 days; then 4 times a day
Vinpocetin	Increases cerebral function; enhances oxygen and glucose production; increases blood flow to circulatory system; beneficial to brain and retinal arteries.	10 mg 3 times a day (If you are on blood-thinning medication or are a hemophiliac, consult your doctor prior to use.)
Huperzine A	Powerful new herbal supplement that enhances memory, focus, and concentration. Studies on AD patients show it is safe and effective long term; protects nerve cells in eyes and ears.	50 mg 2 times a day
DMAE	Elevates mood; promotes restful sleep; increases mental focus, clarity of thought, and muscle tone; may slow age-spot formation on skin and in brain; successfully treats learning disorders in children.	250 mg daily
Acetyl-L-Carnitine (ALC)	Improves memory and learning; improves cerebral blood flow; alleviates depression; elevates mood; at cellular level restores mitochondrial membrane function and membrane fluidity.	250–2000 mg daily

NOOTROPIC	FUNCTION	DAILY DOSE
Phosphatidylserine	Improves cognitive function such as memory, learning, concentration and vocabulary skills; enhances mood, alertness, sociability, and protection from stress.	300 mg 1–3 times a day
Ginkgo Biloba (should contain minimum 24 percent ginkgo flavonglycosides and 6.5 percent terpenes)	Antioxidant, circulation-promoting, daily memory-enhancing properties; fights peripheral vascular insufficiency affecting vision, hypertension, angina, and impaired cerebral flow.	60–240 mg a day
Pregnenolone (a direct precursor of both DHEA and progesterone)	The building block for all other steroidal hormones. Levels decline after age 30, adversely affecting mental function, mood, and energy. Restores these to youthful levels.	100 mg in the A.M.
Coenzyme Q10 (CoQ10)	Causes across-the-board health benefits; positively affects cardiovascular and periodontal health.	60–300 mg split into A.M. and P.M. doses
Lipoic acid	Directly quenches free radicals. Preventive and therapeutic against cataracts, diabetes, heart disease, nerve degeneration, liver disease, and AIDS.	100 mg 2 times daily with meals
SAMe (s-adenosyl-methionine)	Acts as an antidepressant and shows promise against AD. Enhances the function of amino acids, hormones, lipids, minerals, and neurotransmitters. Is found in almost every body tissue.	200 mg 2 times a daily
Glutathione	An important antioxidant defense, *but cannot be absorbed when taken by mouth.*	
N-acetyl-cysteine (*NAC*)	Is easily absorbed from the gut and significantly increases your body's production of brain-protective *glutathione.* Vitamins C and E enhance this effect.	750 mg daily

NOOTROPICS BY PRESCRIPTION

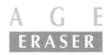

The previously listed nootropics are available without prescription from your favorite food supplement store. The following are available only by prescription from a competent physician.

NOOTROPIC	FUNCTION	DAILY DOSE
Selegiline (*Eldepryl, Deprenyl*)	Enhances mental function; protects neurons; slows AD; inhibits MAO-B that breaks down the neurotransmitter called *dopamine*.	5 mg in A.M.
Piracetam	Mechanism of action is uncertain; reported to have significant memory-enhancing effects. More is *not* better.	Must be adjusted and monitored by physician.
Hydergine (*ergolide mesylate*)	Ergot derivative with potent memory-preserving properties; may be effective in *early* AD.	1–3 mg daily
Dilantin (*diphenylhydantoin*)	Common anticonvulsant used to treat epilepsy and convulsive disorders; stabilizes electrical activity at nerve cell membrane; increases intelligence, concentration, and learning.	25–50 mg daily

eight
antioxidants against
the diseases of aging

Aging can best be described as a process in which the body gradually loses its healthy, functioning cells.

As we age, our bodies produce more and more oxidative agents called *free radicals*. These highly active free radicals literally "crust and rust" your cells. Free radicals are a highly reactive molecule, atom, or molecule fragment that has a free or unpaired electron. Free radicals react quickly with protein, fat, and carbohydrates in the body. They are capable of reacting within almost any cell or tissue and causing a great deal of damage.

They create uncontrolled oxidation that weakens and destroys our cells and lead us to diseases and the very unnatural state of aging. This is caused by oxidation in and around our cells. Just like rust on a bicycle left out in the rain, or an apple left on the counter, the cell deteriorates and is destroyed. Problems occur when free radical production begins to exceed your body's ability to protect against them. This was not happening during your growth and formative years as a child. As an adult, the pendulum swings the other way. The accumulation of free radicals is a part of many disease processes.

Free radicals either destroy the cells through suffocation or severely limit their activity and production. Ultimately, your body's cells lose their ability to regenerate and to provide your organs with the healthy tissue required for proper functioning. One by one, the cellular walls break down, the battle is lost, and aging begins.

I compare this unfortunate process to a beautiful fairway with lush green grass that is thriving with plentiful nutrients and drenched with fresh rainwater and long days of sunshine. As time goes by, the nutrients are depleted, the water dries up, and, one by one, the blades of grass turn brown and wither until finally the beautiful green field has become brown and barren with no life at all.

In your body, a similar process weakens your cells, organs, glands, and tissues, creating a breeding ground for the diseases most commonly associated with aging: cancer, heart disease, arthritis, diabetes, osteoporosis, Alzheimer's disease—millions of us know the list all too well. These diseases prey on weakened, decaying cells and diminished, under-performing immune systems.

RUSTPROOF YOUR CELLS WITH ANTIOXIDANTS

AGE
ERASER

Let's say you've decided to take the advice in this book, and you are going to provide your body with a high-octane energy diet, plenty of fresh water, herbs, nutrients, and minerals. You want to make certain that they can be absorbed and utilized by your cells.

Like a grocery store, your cells need to receive fresh supplies every single day—fresh fruits, meats, and vegetables. What if the trucks that brought the store fresh food found the loading docks blocked and the doors locked? What if the grocery store did not receive fresh supplies each day—what if all that this store had was food that was spoiling or getting rancid? You wouldn't buy your food there, would you?

What does this have to do with your body and antioxidants? It's a way of reminding you that your cells are like that grocery store. Your cells are the providers of the very life that you live day in and day out.

The quality that those cells produce for you will determine the quality of your life, and if they get rancid, spoiled, and overcome with free radicals, they will stop putting out quality. They will stop regenerating energy and they will stop doing their duties. Eventually they will die, and you will start to age rapidly.

Worse yet, once all of this transpires, you can't even bring in the savior—the truck that comes to bring the quality food to the store. The protein, the complex carbohydrates, the minerals and vitamins, the herbs that you so responsibly consumed, will never get into your cells if they are caked and lined with all of these free radicals. The loading docks to your cells will be blocked and locked, and the cells will die from starvation.

Clearly, in order to keep your cells young and healthy you need a powerful ally—antioxidants. Antioxidants are the good guys. They come in the form of enzymes, amino acids, minerals, and vitamins. They protect your body from the bad guys—the free radicals in the black hats that come in and shoot up our cells, putting holes in everything, burning down buildings, and destroying everything you've worked your entire life to build.

Antioxidants are molecular compounds in vitamins and other forms that come in and literally clean away the free radicals that surround the cell. They are nutrients that stop fats, primarily polyunsaturated fatty acids and lipids, from undergoing auto-oxidation or the process of lipid peroxidation.

Owing to their catalytic nature, only low concentrations of nutritional antioxidants are required relative to the oxidizable substrates they protect. I take numerous antioxidants, but, except for Vitamin C, I take each at relatively low levels.

The important point is to take a *complete array of antioxidants* because they work synergistically; each makes the others work to maximum efficiency. Taking them in isolation is like owning all the bricks to build a building without the mortar to hold them together. These antioxidants all work synergistically together. The body has to work harmoniously in balance. You need to take the family of antioxidants.

Antioxidants act catalytically to prevent this oxidative harm. In other words, they speed up chemical reactions without entering into the reaction. They heal the edges of the cell, cleanse it, and open up the loading docks so that you may now feed these cells the nutrients they need to regenerate and energize your life.

Antioxidants are a key component in your quest to remain Forever

Young. If you are going to practice any of the age erasers in this book from hormone replacement to live cell therapy to stimulators of memory and cognitive awareness, your cells must be in condition to accept these nutrients and make use of them. None of it will work if you have filthy, clogged cells that nothing can permeate.

Like a painter, who before applying his craft must scrape off the dry, peeling paint and corrosion, antioxidants scrape the cells clean, allowing them to breathe and to thrive. If there is a St. Peter that literally opens the gates to your cells, it is antioxidants.

Antioxidants come in many sizes, shapes, and forms. The good news is that while there are powerful new supplements and antioxidant formulas introduced every day, some of the most powerful antioxidants come in familiar, pleasant, and inexpensive packages such as orange juice and cruciferous, green, leafy vegetables.

I'm going to give you a short tour of the antioxidants that are part of my life, starting with my favorite. As many of you know, I accompany all of my morning supplements with a tall glass of orange juice.

DRINK A GLASS OF ORANGE JUICE EVERY DAY

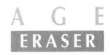

Viewers of my show know that I believe the best way to stay young is to make healthy lifestyle changes that are easy, even pleasurable. I can think of no better example of the "pleasure principle" route to youthfulness than orange juice.

Many of you probably drink orange juice two or three times a week. You enjoy the taste and you've known for some time that Vitamin C is a good thing. But new scientific evidence indicates that the health benefits of orange juice are even more profound. I pour a glass or two of orange juice every single day—and I never miss a day. In fact, after I take a few deep breaths of oxygen in the morning, it's my first "antiaging" activity. I recommend that you do the same thing if you are serious about a lifestyle that helps you stay younger longer.

Folate in Orange Juice Can Help Reduce the Risk of Heart Disease

Most baby boomers, especially women, know about the importance of calcium in their diets. But many may not know that folate is just as important in preserving your good health. A new study from researchers at the University of Florida indicates that folate, which is abundant in orange juice, plays a key role in reducing an important risk factor for heart disease in older women.

In a 14-week study, 33 postmenopausal women, ages 63 to 85, consumed a folate-rich diet consisting of orange juice and foods fortified with folic acid. The diet contained 400 micrograms of folate, which is the recommended daily level. The study showed that these folate foods significantly decreased the levels of homocysteine, a key risk factor for heart disease—the number-one killer of postmenopausal women.

In another study, this one performed by researchers at the Harvard School of Public Health and published in the *Journal of the American Medical Association (JAMA)*, found that a higher consumption of fruits and vegetables, particularly citrus fruits, orange juice, and cruciferous vegetables, corresponded with a substantially reduced risk—up to 30 percent—of ischemic stroke, the most common form of stroke. The Harvard researchers found that drinking a glass of orange juice or grapefruit juice, by itself, lowers your risk of stroke by 25 percent. Researchers speculate that because of its high concentration of fruit, orange juice appeared to be particularly effective in reducing the risk of stroke. One serving typically contains two or three oranges.

Why is this research so significant for those of us who want to remain Forever Young? Stroke is the third leading cause of death and a leading cause of serious disability in the United States. Each year, approximately 700,000 Americans suffer from stroke, and nearly 160,000 Americans die from it. If you can reduce your chances of being part of these sad statistics by 25 percent by simply drinking a glass of orange juice each day, it is wonderful news for anyone who wants to stay healthy and active longer.

Increased Vitamin C Recommendations

In addition to folate, the daily glass of orange juice that you are going to drink has more ways to contribute to your health and vitality—including being the most efficient source of Vitamin C. In April 2000, the National Academy of Sciences (NAS) recommended that Americans increase their daily intake of Vitamin C. The new NAS recommendation is 75 mg daily for women and 90 mg per day for men. The previous recommendation of 60 mg per day had been untouched for 20 years. These levels were set to prevent Vitamin C deficiency. However, in recent years, researchers have studied Vitamin C's role as an antioxidant with the ability to reduce the risks of chronic diseases, including cancer and heart disease.

Throughout this book, I urge you to consume antioxidants. Anyone who follows my television show knows that I believe antioxidants are the singular most important age-management nutrients. And Vitamin C is certainly the "granddaddy" of antioxidants. So it is alarming to me that a third of Americans consume inadequate levels of Vitamin C.

Again, the answer is so deliciously simple. One 10-ounce glass of orange juice provides 100 percent of the new Vitamin C recommendation for men and for women. So put away those tiny orange juice glasses that only give you 4–5 ounces. Bring out your big tumblers and fill them to the brim. Don't settle for less than the full 10 ounces. The health rewards are too important.

Fill Your Glass with Potassium and Phytochemicals Too

You know that I love win-win situations when it comes to health and fitness. Orange juice presents a win-win-win-win scenario. In addition to folate and Vitamin C, orange juice is an excellent source of potassium and phytochemicals.

In fact, a glass of orange juice provides as much potassium as the most famous source of potassium—the banana. Each glass gives you 473 mg of potassium, 25 percent of what the FDA recommends each day. It's a good idea to drink a glass of orange juice each day, and peel yourself a banana too, because potassium plays a key role in lowering blood pressure, which decreases the risk of both heart attacks and strokes, while also regulating heart rhythm.

Orange juice also provides an array of phytochemicals that occur naturally in many fruits and vegetables. According to the nutritionists at the National Cancer Institute, these phytochemicals contribute to the protection of your cells from cancer and other chronic diseases.

If some cutting-edge company were to suddenly discover a new nutrient that had rich amounts of folate, Vitamin C, potassium, and phytochemcials; if they could show clinical studies that proved it could substantially reduce the risk of cancer and heart disease; if they could make it taste delicious and refreshing—the company's stock would double overnight and people would rush to their doctor's office for a prescription. I find it remarkable that all of this health and nutrition exists in something as familiar and inexpensive as a glass of juice. *All we have do is enjoy it every day.*

Remember, I said that staying Forever Young was important. I never said that it always had to be difficult!

VITAMIN C

First, let's review the key component in orange juice, Vitamin C. Vitamin C is a very powerful antioxidant. It plays a primary role in the formation of collagen, which is very important for the growth and repair of tissue, including gums, blood vessels, bones, teeth. It heals wounds, reduces blood cholesterol, and builds the immune system. It dissolves blood clots, helps hold proteins together, and extends the life of Vitamin E. It reduces the negative effects of many allergies and can help lower blood pressure.

VITAMIN A AND CAROTENOIDS

Vitamin A builds resistance to respiratory infections. It aids in the proper function of the immune system. It will shorten the duration of many diseases. It will keep the outer layers of your tissues and organs healthy. It can help in the removal of age spots. Vitamin A and carotenoids are part of Retinol or Retin A that the FDA has approved, and has shown through long-term studies that if applied topically for 18 to 20 months, can reduce wrinkles and remove age spots. That works from the outside in. These products are effective, but I believe in cutting the tree down the other way. You need to do it from the inside out. Just imagine if you put enough Vitamin A inside your body in the proper amounts. Beta-carotene is the best-known carotenoid, but lutein and lycopene are also key. They can be found in many fruits and vegetables, as well as supplements.

VITAMIN E

Vitamin E is one of the most important vitamins on the entire chart. It's fat soluble and is stored in the liver, the heart muscles, the testes, the uterus, in blood, and the adrenal, and pituitary glands. Since we count so much on those glands for our energy and our hormone production and so many other vital functions, the protective qualities of Vitamin E are invaluable to age management. Vitamin E is the most direct antioxidant warrior, attacking free radicals. It is a vasodilator, and an anticoagulant. It keeps you looking younger by retarding cellular aging owed to oxidation. It helps prevent the formation of "bad" cholesterol. It supplies oxygen to your body to give you more endurance. It protects your lungs from pollution. It helps to dissolve blood clots, helps alleviate fatigue, and helps reduce scar tissue. It accelerates healing of burns.

Some scientists believe Vitamin E may even decrease the risk of Alzheimer's disease. I'm amazed that the recommended daily allowance (RDA) recommendations are relatively low. I take a lot more than the RDA. You should determine for yourself the optimum level. Consult your physician to find the best level for you.

SELENIUM

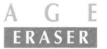

Selenium and Vitamin E are directly synergistic; each one increases the potency of the other. Both slow the aging and hardening of tissue. Selenium is also critical for the production of glutathione peroxidase, which is a primary antioxidant found in every single cell of the human body. Most males have a greater need for selenium. Almost half of their body's supply is concentrated in the testicles and in ducts near the prostate gland. Selenium is lost in semen, so each time the male ejaculates, much of the selenium is lost. Scientists believe that selenium protects against cancer, heart disease, and stroke. It helps eliminate hot flashes and menopausal distress. It helps keep youthful elasticity in the skin, and it can raise the sperm count and fertility in men.

GLUTATHIONE

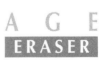

This is a triple powerful antioxidant produced in the liver from three separate amino acids—cysteine, glutamic acid, and glycine. I call this antioxidant "Mr. Clean" because of the power it has to truly cleanse your cells. Glutathione protects cells throughout the body as well as all organ tissue. It may actually help prevent cancer, especially of the liver. Remember, glutathione is in each cell in the human body. It functions as an immune-system booster, a detoxifier of heavy metals and drugs, and may protect against the detrimental effects of radiation, cigarette smoke, and alcohol. It is an anti-inflammatory, and is often used in the treatment of arthritis and allergies. It is found in many fruits and vegetables, but cooking reduces its potency, so I suggest supplementing the diet. I take 200 mg per day of this powerful antioxidant.

MANGANESE

Manganese helps activate the enzymes necessary for the body's proper use of several B vitamins and Vitamin C. It is needed for normal bone structure in the body and is important for the formation of thyroxin, the principal hormone of the thyroid gland. It is also important for the reproduction of the central nervous system and proper digestion and utilization of foods. It can help eliminate fatigue and keeps your energy levels at a much higher level. It aids in muscle reflexes, especially if you work out a lot. It helps in the battle against osteoporosis, one of the most common aging diseases. It is said to improve memory and nervous irritability. It is necessary to produce the antioxidant enzyme superoxide dismutase (SOD). This helps revitalize skin tissue cells and reduce the rate of cell destruction. As we age, our bodies produce less and less SOD, so the supplementation of manganese, which helps your body create it (or SOD directly), becomes an important factor in the reduction of wrinkles and retarding the aging process on all levels. I take three to four supplements every single morning, in the form of wheat grass.

CYSTINE AND CYSTEINE

Cystine is the stable form of the sulfer-containing amino acid cysteine—an important antiaging nutrient. The body readily converts the former into the latter when needed. When cystine is metabolized, it yields sulfuric acid, which reacts with other substances that help detoxify the system. It is especially important to protect and restore cells among smokers and drinkers of alcohol. It can be easily taken in supplement form, L-cysteine. Its protective effects are especially significant in tandem with Vitamin C.

METHIONINE

This is a powerful antioxidant that helps break down fats in the body. It helps protect the body from various toxins and free radicals. When combined with choline and folic acid, it has been shown to offer protection against certain tumors. It also helps women with the secretion of estrogen. A methionine deficiency has been linked to cholesterol deposits, atherosclerosis, and hair loss in laboratory animals. An insufficiency can lead to edema and infection. It is not synthesized in the body, so must be obtained from food and supplements. Good food sources of this amino acid are beans, fish, eggs, garlic, soybeans, meat, onions, seeds, and yogurt.

COENZYME Q10

CoQ10 has received a great deal of recognition and publicity recently. While it has a rather exotic sounding name, it is a basic antioxidant nutrient that is found in every living cell. It is essential in providing your cells with the energy necessary for your body to carry out its activities. As we age, levels of CoQ10 fall, which may directly relate to numerous diseases and illness associated with aging. It is very important to proper cardiovascular function and a healthy heart. It has also been shown to increase energy, help reverse gum disease, and improve the immune system. It is found in meat, cereals, vegetables, eggs, and dairy products—but cooking and processing deplete it, so supplementation is important. It is expensive, so shop around for the best value.

PYCNOGENOL

Pycnogenol is comprised of varous forms of bioflavonoids extracted from the bark of French pine trees. It is perhaps France's greatest gift to the United States since the Statue of Liberty. It acts as a potent anti-inflammatory agent, reducing inflammation linked to arthritis, varicose veins, and numerous allergies, by inhibiting the release of enzymes that cause swelling. It protects skin by stabilizing collagen, the abundant protein in the skin. It improves skin smoothness and elasticity by strengthening tiny capillaries that deliver the blood to nourish cells. It also offers protection against the ultraviolet rays of the sun that lead to skin cancer.

REMEMBER TO GET THE COMPLETE FAMILY OF ANTIOXIDANTS

According to a pioneer in antioxidant research, Dr. Richard Passwater, "Combinations of antioxidants are like a balanced symphony working together. A symphony orchestra produces sounds so much more harmonious than merely having 20 drums playing. It is not the quantity, but the blend. The same is true of antioxidants. You will get far better results with moderate amounts of a full complement than you get by using very large amounts of one nutrient. If you take large quantities of Vitamin E in the absence of selenium, Vitamin C, and carotenoids, that would be far less effective in your body than taking 200 mg of Vitamin E and Vitamin C, plus 10 or 20 mg of carotenoids and 200 mg of selenium."

I agree 100 percent with Dr. Passwater's observations. It is not the *quantity* but the *blend*. The reason my company puts the formula of antioxidants together in our age-management formula is that they are all synergistically compatible and they go so far in maximizing the performance of all of the other vitamins, minerals, and herbs that are in that formula. I know that not everyone is going to be like me and carry suitcases full of vitamins, minerals, and herbs everywhere they go, so we put a balanced and complete blend in this product. Check my web site, **www.BillFranksForeverYoung.com**, for more information.

nine turbocharge your
energy levels

From time to time people tell me that when I'm on, I can electrify a room. They say I really light it up. This may be because I don't live a day without trying to be highly energized.

I tell you this not to boast, but to begin the story of how to unleash amazing levels of energy in your life—levels that I believe we are all intended to have. In the next few pages, I'm going to tell you about a wealth of exercises, vitamins, herbs, hormones, and antioxidants that will give your energy level a remarkable boost. I'm going to tell you about new techniques to give you youthful vitality and exuberance that you probably haven't felt for decades.

But first, I want to remind you that all energy has a source, a point of origin. And I can tell you that it all starts inside of you—in your heart and in your mind. Even if you don't read another chapter in this book, you will have gotten your money's worth if you learn to generate and harness the energy in your life. Because energy is *youth*, and energy is *life*.

On those days when I "light it up" I walk in with purpose. More often than not, I have a mission in mind—a plan of what I want to accomplish. That's the way I try to approach my whole life.

I don't know about you, but I like to have my presence felt. I like people to be happier, more motivated, and more full of life because I walked into that room. I like to share my energy and give it away. Because the wonderful part about this kind of energy is that when you give it away, you don't have to give it up. In fact, you usually get *more* back. So I walk in with visualization—a plan of what I want to accomplish, and the decision that I might as well have some fun doing it!

Think about your day. Why not go out there and give it everything you've got? Put a little showmanship into it. Go in with a positive attitude and a smile on your face. Go in with exuberance and a high energy level. Speak with a vibrant quality in your voice. Let them see that smiling face! Let them see those eyes sparkle!

The message coming from inside of you, whatever that message may be, must be delivered with power and energy. It is so easy to believe someone who is confidant and full of life. It is so difficult to believe someone who barely whispers, speaks timidly to you about something, and just has no energy. They're lifeless. You just want to run and hide. They're the ones who put you to sleep.

These people speak in a monotone; there is no energy. They contribute nothing to your day except to put you to sleep for 30 or 40 minutes. These are not people who are motivating others. They are not delivering their message. Their heart is just not in it. And the simple ingredient that is missing is energy.

When you put your heart into life, energy follows. Anyone who is committed to accomplishment knows that if you cannot do it with dynamic energy and audacity you are not going to get the job done. So once you believe in you, and once you know that you are going to call upon your body to perform, your brain has done its part. Your emotional state has done its part. Now it's time to make sure that your body does its part too.

You are not meant to be sluggish, tired, and run-down. You are not meant to become a tired old man or woman. You are meant to operate like the finest Indianapolis 500 engine ever built and you are made to operate for all 500 miles—not a few laps, not a couple hundred miles. You are designed to go 500 miles and beyond.

As human beings, we are designed to live well over a century of life. If we feel tired and exhausted and tapped out, we do it to ourselves. We are not aging rapidly when we are at a high energy level. People see individuals who are very active and say, "Oh, they're burning themselves out." But it is the couch potatoes who are burning themselves out! The person who is full of stress in life and does not want to do anything about it except whine and complain and cry to somebody else—that's a candidate for burnout. No, the energized bunny, the one who goes on and on and on, is going to stay younger longer.

I am never so tired as when I have just gone shopping. Over the years, I found that when I went shopping I would move so slowly that I just wanted to go to sleep by the time I'd finished. I was doing just enough movement for my body to be producing lactic acid. I was doing just enough movement for fatigue products to bounce around and get in my bloodstream and make me feel like I didn't want to do anything but take a nap. I'd want to hit the couch, put my feet up, and take a snooze. I know most of you can identify with this feeling. However, it is just these moments that afford you the opportunity to begin to make your Forever Young lifestyle changes. It is now more than ever that you must realize just how quickly active exercise of any kind can reverse this feeling.

When the battery in your car goes dead, you don't just let it sit there. If you do, it's dead and it's always going to be dead. So instead, you jump-start it. And then you charge it by running it down the highway. You make it work. You use it. You go 50 miles down the road until you have a completely recharged battery. But how can it really be recharged? It was dead an hour ago. No, you just *thought* it was dead. It was dying from inactivity or the wrong kind of activity. It was full of sludge. *The sludge just needed to be worked out and the battery cells recharged.*

You will never *over*work. You will only *under*work. You won't *over*exercise; you'll *under*exercise. Now that doesn't mean that I'm

turbocharge your
energy levels

going to send you on a 24-hour marathon. But I *am* going to tell you that when you feel you're too tired to work out, that's often exactly what you need to do!

I like to move blood from the top of my head to the tip of my toes and back around again. That's cardiovascular and I can do that with weights as well as by running on a treadmill or stepping on a Stairmaster. But I go at a high intensity level. I want all of my energy to be focused on the body part that I am working. I want to concentrate on sending blood into my chest area, then into my back, into my shoulders and into my arms. I want to be like a charged engine that's moving blood throughout my body.

I want to cleanse my body of all the lactic acids and the fatigue products that have built up. I want to wash out my body and be left with nothing but the positive feeling that I have energized muscle. I have new nitrogen in it. I'm hydrated. I'm all pumped up and I'm really ready to go.

Sometimes when I'm working in my office and have done a lot of reading or have been to one meeting after another, someone will tell me I look tired and recommends that I get some rest. I'm sure that's happened to you too. But here's where you make the change! Just say, "You're right, I need to get out of here for a while." Then go to the gym, take a power walk, do anything *except* get some rest. When you go back to work and people say, "Boy, you look great! See, I told you that you needed to get out of here," just give them a great big smile and say, "You're right!"

A G E ERASER

LIVE WITH VIGOR

I can tell you that the correlation between living a vigorous life and living a long and healthy life is absolute. Before I was known for my staying Forever Young advice, my clients in major league baseball gave me the name "Vigor Man."

At that time I had developed a product called Body Vigor, and I was drinking it all of the time and passing it on to them. Many of the high-energy vitamins, herbs, minerals, and antioxidants that I recommend in this chapter were in Body Vigor.

But what really got them was that I would go to spring training and they would start seeing me at 7:00 in the morning hitting balls with them, doing laps, running drills, goofing off, and having fun—just like a kid at the playground. What further surprised them was that they would still see me at 9:00 or 10:00 in the evening and my behavior pattern was the very same. They knew that I hadn't taken any nap—I had been with them all day long.

So we were both expending an enormous amount of energy, and they kept wondering how I could keep up with them day in and day out. They would say, "Show us how you do it, Vigor Man." And that's exactly what I did. Guys like Nolan Ryan, Ozzie Smith, Dave Parker, Donny Baylor, Brian Downing—I showed how to supercharge their energy levels, elevate their games, and extend their playing days.

Although the information has been updated, the rest of this chapter will teach you what I taught them about putting more vitality and energy in their lives. Once you decide that you are going to live with vigor, the rest is simply mechanics.

USE HIGH-ENERGY FUEL, WITH NO ENERGY ZAPPERS

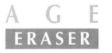

Before I even start to talk about what to put in your body, I have to remind you what to keep out. Here's what I do (or don't do). I try not to let any energy zappers in. Most of the time, I keep alcohol out of my body. Occasionally, I will drink a nice glass of wine or a good brandy. I allow myself just one cup of coffee each day during the week, and I refrain on the weekends. I certainly don't smoke or do anything to deny myself the precious oxygen my body needs to transmit fuel and energy throughout my body. I very rarely indulge in fast food, junk food, soda pop, sugar, salt, or artificial sweeteners—you know the list. I try not to do any of the things that will interrupt the energy flowing from my brain, to my neurotransmitters, to my muscles and cells. I want good carbohydrates to go into my body—not empty ones. I don't want a lot of starches. I want fresh vegetables and fruits going into my body, providing just enough glucose to energize it and make it want to get active.

As I mentioned in the chapters about losing fat and gaining muscle, carbohydrates ought to comprise 30 percent of your caloric intake. If you are going to be active, you want the complex carbohydrates to energize you, whether you're out there to run, jog, lift weights, or to play tennis, golf, or basketball.

Protein is also critical to energy conversion. In Plan B, the 60 percent I recommend for fat loss and physique building is just as important for creating a peak energy level. Nitrogen is the cellular regenerator in the human body. It is converted from protein. This conversion is the starting point for all cellular activity, and must be working at optimum levels to enhance the flow of energy into your muscle tissue. As your muscles increase in density, your metabolism increases and you have more energy at your body's beck and call.

Let's assume that with this extra energy you're going to engage in more physical activity. This will feed the energy cycle, and you'll have even more. Your body will be glad it has the advantage of a lot of protein. As the years roll by on your knees, elbows, ankles, and hips—the joints required to move you around—they must be supported with lean muscle tissue. The same holds true of the transmitters in the vertebrae in your spine. You want lean muscle mass around them to support them and to lessen the burden they must bear as you get older. So you must keep a strong protein/nitrogen balance in your body. Load yourself up with good quality protein. This means lean meats, chicken, and fish, especially from clean, fresh water. If you are one of those who believe you should not eat egg yolks, then just eat the whites. Personally, I believe that eggs have taken an unfair beating. An egg is one of the finest sources of protein on the planet. It is the perfect food. It is an absolutely magnificent food. I know many individuals who have eaten several eggs almost every day of their lives and they don't have a cholesterol problem.

"SMART" FATS WILL ENERGIZE YOUR DIET

Now that you have created the nutritional building blocks for efficient energy conversion, the next step toward boundless energy is managing the fats in your diet. You want the fats that you allow in your body to be essential fatty acids. Stay away from greasy fats—the bacon and sausage and cheeseburger variety that literally coat your cells and prevent them from getting any nitrogen. Think about it. Do you ever feel anything but lethargic an hour or so after a visit to your neighborhood fast food establishment for a super-deluxe bacon cheeseburger?

Essential fatty acids (EFAs) are dietary fats and oils that have a mentally and physically positive influence on you. Your heart needs a certain amount of these "smart" fats, as they are called. You need linolenic acid

(LA), gama linolenic acid (GLA), eicosapentaenoic acid (EPA), docosapentaenoic acid (DPA), and docosahexaenoic acid (DHA).

Fish lipids (supplements made from fat found in fish) and flaxseed provide some of the best sources of omega-3 fatty acids. They are EFAs that:

➤ Help fight high blood pressure, inflammation, and water retention
➤ Increase overall function of the cardiovascular system
➤ Aid in increasing nerve and brain function
➤ Lower blood triglycerides and cholesterol levels

Borage oil and black currant seed are GLAs. GLAs are part of the omega 6 series of EFAs. GLAs are normally synthesized in the liver from dietary linolenic acid (LA). In a large part of the U.S. population, excess sugar consumption interferes with this process. GLA is a critical precursor to the series 1 prostaglandins (PGE1) and other hormones in our bodies. The PGE1 protect the body against the damaging effects of the PGE2 prostaglandin series, which include:

➤ High blood pressure
➤ Inflammation
➤ Sticky platelets
➤ Lowered immune system
➤ Water retention

The PGE2 series are a result of arachidonic acid created by overconsumption of animal products. Notice I said *over*consumption—not normal consumption.

Keep your fats coming from the linolenic acids (LAs), the alpha linolenic acids (ALAs), the GLAs, and the EPAs. These are the fats that you want to keep in your body to support your heart, brain, skin, muscles, and cells. Essential fatty acids help keep your cells clean, which is a must for this finely tuned race car you want to build for energy conversion and utilization.

A Quick Summary

Omega-3 essential fatty acids are considered alpha linolenic acids. They come in things like flax, flaxseed oil, pumpkin seeds, chai, and walnuts.

California walnuts are a great way to get the omega-3s. I buy them by the bag and eat roughly a handful a day. Keep them handy in the refrigerator for a convenient snack any time. It's much healthier than a cookie or a piece of candy, and it will give you a little shot of energy. Essential fatty acids are an important part of your body's energy production machine, because they help create activity, starting in the brain and then sending energizing signals throughout your body.

The omega-6 fatty acids are the linolenic acids, which are oils from corn, safflower, sunflower, and sesame seeds.

EPA is found in cold-water fish and algae from certain parts of the world. EPA stands for *eicosapentaenoic acid*. The creator of that particular name wanted to be sure that you never forgot him! It is a long-chain polyunsaturated fatty acid derived from dietary alpha linolenic acid. It is an anti-inflammatory substance that reduces cholesterol, lubricates joints, softens skin, and enhances brain function. GLAs are the oils from primrose, borage, and black currant seed.

If your diet does not contain adequate essential fatty acids, the intestinal membranes will also not contain adequate amount of EFAs. Rebuilding of the body will be difficult because you will not extract the nutrients from the foods that you need to nourish the cells. Absorption of the nutrients is very important. You must constantly repair the intestinal walls and the cells inside them. They require the linolenic acids, GLAs, ALAs, and EPAs for proper cell building.

When you combine 10 percent fatty acids, 30 percent carbohydrates, and 60 percent lean protein with exercise, you will have a smooth-running, efficient power plant for energy. This is the formula that will constantly fuel your body's regeneration process. Muscle activity gets it all started and then this ideal combination of nutrients goes to work. This keeps the body pure and clean and keeps it running like a perfectly tuned engine, churning out energy like you've never felt before.

For the exercise part of the program, I prefer to lift weights and supplement with tennis, golf, track, and everything else. In my chapter on cycling and training, I explain to you why I prefer weight training as the central focus of my particular fitness program. You may prefer to do circuit training or emphasize aerobics. Whatever your choice, just try to do it two or three hours every week.

You have heard "Lean is mean," "Stay thin," and all of these phrases, but many times we do that at the cost of muscle mass. What the world considers *normal* is that as you age your muscle mass is going to decrease. You start thinning out. You start losing muscle tone. It is my belief that you should do whatever you can to keep as much muscle mass on your body as you can, for as long as you can. More lean muscle mass in your body will elevate your metabolism and your energy output. It will also help protect you against the early onset of osteoporosis and other degenerative diseases that attack our bone and joint structure. In addition, this is an amazing energy-generating process, which you can harness if you incorporate this formula into your life.

KEEP SLEEP PATTERNS CONSTANT

When it comes time to lie down at night at whatever hour is your normal bedtime, make it constant. Remember, the body operates in rhythms and cycles. If your normal sleep cycle is 10:00 at night until 6:00 the next morning, make it a habit. Don't change it on the weekends and throw your system out of whack just because it's the weekend and you think you should sleep in. Get up! Live your life the same way every day when it comes to your sleep pattern. This will keep your energy flowing at its maximum levels.

If you are an eight-hour sleeper, then you are an eight-hour sleeper. However, there are those in the medical profession who will tell you that if you are a ten-hour sleeper, you are getting closer to the grave every day because you are sleeping your life away, and I agree with them. There is such a thing as too much sleep as an adult. I am not going to tell you how much sleep you need. But I am going to tell you that ten hours is too much and four hours is too little for most people.

Somewhere in the range of six to eight hours is where your body will regenerate and recuperate. I like to change my routine when it comes to exercise and food. But sleep is different. Sleep is your body's time to recover. Giving recovery a specific, unchanging time and place will optimize the efficiency and results so that each day you can wake up and thank the creator that you have another day to go out and conquer. "I feel great!" Remember, you want a *grrrrreat* so great that Tony the Tiger will take lessons from you.

EXUDE THE RIGHT KIND OF ENERGY

In many ways, each of us is a self-contained universe that generates and releases energy into the rest of the world. Are we giving off positive energy or are we giving off negative energy? In many cases, we are either taking energy away from somebody or we are giving energy to somebody. Think about the people in your personal or business life. I'll bet you can fit most of them into one category or the other.

In my life, I have found that energy is much like love. The more love I give away, the more comes my way. The more energy I throw out into the world, the more I seem to receive in return. The well seems to never ever go dry. As I sit here writing at 12:30 A.M., my legs are moving up and down a mile a minute. I'm not hyperactive, I just have a lot of energy because I'm so excited about writing this book. I could just as easily be taking my dumbbells off the rack and working out, because I have all of this incredible flow of energy. What are you doing when you feel the most energized? Preparing for a big meeting? Coaching a Little League team? Preparing for a dinner party? I'm willing to bet it's not when you're preparing your taxes or driving to the dentist.

The more time that you can spend in activities that empower and satisfy you, the more you are going to be throwing positive energy out into the world. Fatigue is not natural. And neither is aging. We allow ourselves to follow these paths because we let our minds lead us there. We age because we are inactive or accept a preconceived notion of what will happen to us. We age because we stop feeling like the little child who is so full of life and wonder.

Energy is simply a state of mind, knowing what you want, knowing how to get it, and backing it up by taking care of your body. That's what this book and all of the age erasers are all about. Once you get the mental picture and decide how good you're going to feel when you achieve it, you will find—or create—all of the energy you need to make it happen. You'll soon be recognized as someone who not only exercises with energy but as someone who enlivens every day for yourself and all of those around you. To that end, here are my top-10 energizers:

1. **Strive for ultimate hydration.** Drink at least ten 12-ounce glasses of water daily. I prefer using distilled water. One day each week fast on only distilled water for 24 hours.

2. **Maintain a consistent sleep cycle of six to eight hours every night.** Stay consistent. Try to go to bed and get up at the same time weekdays and weekends.

3. **Begin each day with 10 to 12 minutes of stretching and flexing exercises.** Stand on your head or use an inversion machine if you have one. Follow the exercises with a shower consisting of 30 seconds of cold water, 60 seconds of hot water, followed by another 30 seconds of cold. This is invigorating!

4. **Start your day with a good breakfast.** Go light on fat, modest on carbohydrates to fuel the engine, and include at least 25–40 g of protein to support your morning activities.

5. **Supplement your breakfast with a well-balanced vitamin and herbal formula.** Minerals should be taken with lunch or dinner. Make sure that your morning supplements contain an adequate (100 mg of most of the B family) amount of B vitamins. Try to find a B supplement that provides approximately 25–50 mg of niacin. Make sure that your formula contains Vitamins A, C, D, and E. (I prefer to save my E to take at bedtime as I find that the oil tends to absorb better during sleep.)

   Individuals have varied reactions to herbs. I encourage you to start with a good ginseng base containing a multiple ginseng formula. By this I mean a formula that contains a combination of American, Siberian Panax, Korean, and even some of the Indian herbs such as ashwaganda. You may also add kola nut, guarana, ginkgo biloba, and schisandra (avoid this if pregnant or if you suffer from high blood pressure).

6. **Take a brisk 10-minute walk *prior to lunch.*** As you walk, remember to breathe well and concentrate on making at least 10 of these (one a minute) really deep breaths drawn in through your nose and exhaled strongly out through your mouth.

7. **Always make lunch a lighter meal than breakfast.** It should be supplemented with herbs such as catawba, muira puama, guarana, damiana, gotu kola, suma (for both men and women), dong quai, chaste berry (for women only), fo-ti-t'eng (for men only), and ginkgo biloba and butcher's broom (for both). This will help you stay alert and awake all afternoon.

8. **Make dinner the lightest meal of the day.** Go heavy on protein, low on fat, and very light on carbohydrates. Do not take energizing herbs with your dinner. You may take primrose, valerian root, bilberry, and Vitamin E at this time.

9. **Hit the gym.** Whatever your routine, whether it is weight lifting three times weekly and/or aerobics three times weekly, burn off your evening meal, cleanse your body, calm your nerves, and lower your blood pressure for a good night's sleep. For those who work a second- or third-shift job, try to exercise first thing in the morning. Try to leave three hours between when you finish exercising and your bedtime.

10. **The most important energizer of all: spend a pleasant, peaceful, harmonious evening with those you love.** This calms all the nerve centers that you've energized throughout the day, and allows all of nature's life forces to regenerate during sleep.

NOTE: *I do not advise using stimulants like ephedra and other thermogenics available as an energizer. They may increase your blood pressure and overstimulate your heart. Try living my 10 energizers and see if they don't make a positive change in your life.*

ten

keeping your sex life young

Unfortunately, the one universally accepted side effect of aging is the reduction of sexuality. Less desire. Less performance. Less satisfaction. How many relationships have been ruined? How many lives have been thrown into depression by this seemingly inevitable slowdown in sexual function?

But is this decline in one of life's most profound pleasures really inevitable? "Of course it is," you say. "Why, even Hugh Hefner is on Viagra!" Well, you know me, I don't accept any aging process as inevitable, certainly not one as precious and important to happiness as sex. We are meant to be able to make love for as long as we want to. There's nothing natural about shutting it off and letting it slow down, and yet we do just that.

Unfortunately, there really is a succession of processes in the body that make the decline in sexual function very real as the years add up. Although the common excuse for lack of desire or performance is "a rough day at the office," according to the National Institutes of Health's consensus panel on impotence, physical causes are responsible for 75 percent of the cases of impotence. In men over 50, the figure is 90 percent.

In many middle-age cases, the culprit isn't age; it is arteriosclerosis of the penile arteries—the same problem that leads to heart disease. Of course, for many men impotence isn't an issue; the problem is a general decline in libido, sexual performance, and satisfaction. It is well documented that women in this age group experience menopause, which may sometimes lead to a decline in libido and sexual enjoyment. It is less known that many middle-aged men experience a similar endocrine-related process called *andropause*, which also leads to the reduction in sexual response. The exciting news is that we now know how to stop and reverse this process.

I'm going to teach you how to physiologically revitalize your sex life. Women can experience greater libido and satisfaction, and men can experience better erections, longer duration, and less recovery time between orgasms.

But first, the bad news: As we age, our internal organs shrink.

Sorry to have to tell you that, but if it's any solace, keep in mind, I said "internal" organs. Let's take a look inside the body of an aging lover. The first thing that happens as he/she moves into the mid-20s is that the endocrine system of hormonal organs—the hypothalamus, the thyroid, and the pituitary gland—begins to decline in size and function.

Less hormones are produced, particularly human growth hormone (hGH). Every decade of your life, production drops off about 14 percent. That means testosterone and estrogen levels decline, as do a host of other hormones that contribute to sexual function. There are only two real explosive hormone growth periods in your life. One is not long after you start walking, between three and four years of age. And, believe it or not, after that it settles down and very little takes place until you hit puberty. Then there's this huge explosion that young adolescents must navigate through. External sexual characteristics appear, and there is enormous growth in internal organs too.

Most people peak at 19 years of age. Some are a little slower, but by age 22 almost everyone has finished producing hormones at peak levels. And then hGH starts slowing down and insulin-like growth factor (IGF) levels are greatly reduced. When they slow down, the organs in your body—the liver, the pancreas, the spleen, the heart—slowly but surely begin to shrink inside your body.

If we are not doing anything to stimulate the system, muscles and bones shrink too. It's true that as we get older, we get shorter. This is a direct result of the fact that the organs that produce all of these hormones are becoming smaller and less efficient. This affects every human response, especially sexuality.

Not a pretty picture. It kind of reminds me of the character in the 1957 science fiction movie *The Incredible Shrinking Man* who spent most of the movie hiding from cats and battling spiders twice his size. I paint this picture not to make you feel small, but to help you understand that these very real declining processes can be stopped and reversed.

DECIDE TO REVERSE DECLINING SEXUALITY

The decline in human sexuality is well documented, and fortunately, so is the ability to reverse it. According to the Kinsey Institute, 2 percent of men under 40 are impotent. By the age of 80, 75 percent of men are incapable of having or sustaining an erection. The Massachusetts Male Aging Study found that incidences of complete erectile dysfunction increased steadily from 5 percent at age 40 to 15 percent at age 79, with difficulty in sustaining erections experienced by 52 percent in the older age group.

Loss of ability to perform is not just a problem for men but, of course, also affects the relationship with the female in their life. Lack of understanding of the problem and its causes by all parties, if gone untreated, can lead to frustration and a resulting loss of intimacy. Add to that the decline of estrogen levels in women with all of its possible side effects— mood swings, hot flashes, depression, and vaginal dryness to mention a few—and you have a potential recipe for trouble in the relationship.

It has been noted by numerous scientists that the loss of sexual desire and performance closely parallels the decline in the function of the endocrine hormones. The first clinical analysis of hormone replacement and sexuality was done by Dr. L. Cass Terry and his associates, the same scientist who wrote Chapter Seven of this book. Dr. Terry found that 75 percent of the participants said that they had an increase in sexual desire and frequency, and 62 percent of the men reported that they were able to maintain an erection for a longer period of time. I'll talk in more detail about various types of hormone interventions later in this chapter, and in even more detail in Chapter Eleven.

The important point here is that there are numerous ways to reverse declining sexuality—including hormones, exercise, diet, vitamins, minerals, and ancient oriental herbs. It's hard to think of a compelling reason not to take advantage of this wonderful new age of information and science, which I will now review.

STIMULATE, STIMULATE, STIMULATE

The first way to reverse this shrinking and declining process is to continuously stimulate the organs. Ironically, just at the age that these organs need incremental stimulation, most of us are providing less. Our lives become more sedentary and our diets become erratic. Stress inhibits these functions even more.

How do you stimulate internal organs? Some of this is done with activity, some through proper nutrition and medicine. The first thing you must do is find ways to produce more human growth hormone (hGH). It is the hormonal granddaddy of everything inside. Even though it's the king of the country, it has to have its court to get things done. That's what the other organs of the body are. The hGH in your body has to drive all of your organs to function at peak levels in order for you to be at your best in any aspect of life, especially your sex life.

Just think of how your body goes to work each time your loved one gives you the right signal or touch. Your heart and lungs are working faster and harder. Your endocrine system—your hypothalamus, your thyroid, your adrenal glands, and your testes or ovaries—are moving hormones through your body at lightning speed. Blood is rushing though your body to all of the important places. All of your body's senses are heightened.

In a young, healthy body, this process works efficiently and smoothly. But if the muscles in your heart are pumping a little weaker, your lungs are oxygenating at lower levels, and if the organs in your endocrine system have declined in size and production, you can see why sexual desire and performance can be diminished.

What's the easiest, most natural way to stimulate all of these processes? The right kind of exercises. It's ironic that just at the time when the aging body requires more exercise to stimulate it, most of us are reaching the point where we are providing it with less.

There are certain exercises you can do that will stimulate additional release of human growth hormone for several hours at a time. A lot of people wonder why, after going to the gym and doing heavy leg presses and squats, or other strenuous leg workout routines, they come home and are easily aroused. This is why:

They're in the mood to make love because their hGH levels are elevated, their testosterone and estradiol levels are pulled right along with it, and they are ready to go. They may not be ready for a marathon because their legs are fatigued, but they are ready to go sexually.

Sex is a process that is driven by blood moving to the right parts of the body. I'm going to teach you some specific exercises that not only will increase the hGH moving through your body, but will increase the flow of blood to exactly the places you want it.

STRENGTHEN YOUR "LOVE MUSCLES" AND KEEP BLOOD FLOWING

Before I get into more complex methods of enhancing sexuality, I'm going to start with the most basic and natural—adding the right kind of physical exertion to your life. There are two times when hormone production is very high in adults: during sexual activity and during extreme muscular exertion or stress. In men, some high-intensity workouts, such as very heavy squats and very heavy dead-lifts, produce high levels of human growth hormone that increases virility and, at the same time, builds muscle and bone density. This leads to enhanced libido and, ultimately, to the pursuit of your sexual partner.

I'll discuss the subject of aphrodisiacs and hormonal supplements later in this chapter, but perhaps the greatest aphrodisiac of all is a fit, firm, healthy partner. Good health and self-discipline are sexy. Conversely, letting yourself go is often contagious and can lead to a spiraling down of sexual desire for both partners. Sex is, of course, a deeply emotional event, but it is also one of the most physical of human drives. Hence, maintaining physical fitness can help you keep a youthful energy and vitality in both your relationship and your sex life.

There are some very basic physiological reasons that people who are well conditioned make better lovers, no matter what their biological age. The body performs in some miraculous ways. Ironically, in an unfit lover, the body may work to make sex more difficult. As soon as any part of the body senses an oxygen deficit, a state of fatigue begins, and blood comes racing to that part of the body.

Usually the heart and lungs are the first recipient of this influx of blood and oxygen, thereby pulling the blood from the sexual zones of the body. A well-conditioned lover will not be nearly as inclined to require this extensive movement of blood through the body—blood moving in the wrong direction for the business at hand.

If you have a lot of excess weight around your abdomen, your circulation will be inhibited and the ability to perform sexually declines. In a man, an erection can utilize from a half to a full pint of blood. That's up to one-seventh of the seven pints that most bodies contain. In a woman, blood needs to reach all of the vital nerve endings in the genital area. If you are overweight and out of condition, fatigue can occur quickly. It's just difficult for your body to get the blood where it needs to be. The blood that is circulating through all that fat around your middle has a difficult time getting where you want it.

On the other hand, if you develop the muscles in the lower regions of your body—your abdomen, your buttocks, your hips, your thighs—you will stimulate muscle development, hormone release, bone development, and circulation, which will enhance sexual performance—assuming, of course, the absence of any prohibiting physical or emotional conditions.

Beyond a good diet, aerobic exercise, and an ongoing weight-resistance program, I recommend some very specific exercises to get the blood flowing and moving to the right places in your body. A 45-year-old male or female who is fit and muscular in these areas of the body has a much better chance of a healthy sex life than a 45-year-old who has let time and a sedentary lifestyle take its course unchecked.

The exercises I recommend to work your body's "love muscles" are squats, barbell curls, heavy bench presses, and military presses. There are photographs and demonstrations of these exercises in Chapter Six. These specific exercises not only help your circulation, they also stimulate the release of hGH in your body, which stimulates your libido and increases your ability to perform sexually.

The exercises I have recommended are one definite way to increase the production and release of hGH in your body. The exercises can directly affect your libido. The release of hGH stimulates an increased release of testosterone. It helps cycle DHEA and all of the other hormones that are so necessary to well-balanced health and youthfulness. hGH also stimulates endorphins in your body, which are part of the chemistry that creates libido.

GOOD HEALTH = GOOD SEX

If you want to prolong a healthy and active sex life, you have to take care of your basic health maintenance behaviors. If the vague promise of good health doesn't always keep you on track, maybe the more narrowly focused promise of being a good sexual partner longer will help you pay attention to some basic healthy habits.

There is a hierarchy of interventions you can make to prolong and enhance your sexual functions. Before you go to the more severe techniques, I recommend starting with the simplest. You would be surprised how many people lose sight of these simple steps, and whose sex lives could get a boost from a collection of some very easy lifestyle changes.

A HEALTHY DINNER IS A ROMANTIC DINNER

Once you've decided to focus on a sexual antiaging plan, go back and read Chapter Three on your antiaging diet. It is an integral part of keeping your sexual life healthy. You must balance your body. In other words, you must have a balance of all of the nutrients in your body—protein, carbohydrates, vitamins, minerals, fats, and water.

If any one of these things is out of whack, it can create an inactive level somewhere in your body. With all of the complex chemistry that happens every time you even think about sex, it is no surprise that this is one area that easily shows the results of dietary imbalance. All of the sugars, salts, fats, and artificial ingredients that I urge you to purge from your diet are the antithesis of creating the environment in your body that leads to fulfilling sex into the middle and later ages of your life. In your 20s and 30s nothing can stop your hormones and sexual response. But as you get into your 40s and beyond, I strongly recommend predisposing your body to healthy functioning in every way you can.

Remember, even the manufacturers of Viagra who recommend it be taken one hour before any sexual activity, recommend that it not be taken for three hours after a meal containing a large amount of fat. This is because they recognize the importance of moving the fat out of the bloodstream so that it doesn't block the vasodilation effects of the drug.

Now, go back and read Chapter Three again if you need to. Implement the first phase of your body's age-management program for your sex life—lose your body fat—and then begin to think about the following more advanced therapies and programs.

MORE ADVANCED PRO-SEXUAL INTERVENTIONS

There are numerous prescription drugs that are considered pro-sexual. They claim to enhance libido for both men and women, to strengthen erections or the ease of erections, to promote longer-lasting erections, and to improve the frequency of orgasms for both sexes. They range from L-dopa, originally a treatment for Parkinson's disease, Bromocriptine, Deprenyl, to GHB or gamma-hydroxybutyrate. All can be used by men or women.

It is not my intent, however, to describe the merits of these prescription drugs in this book. Ask your physician to take the time to give you his or her opinion of any of the above as they relate to your particular condition, situation, and health goals.

I will, however, describe some of the natural nutrients and hormonal supplements that will affect libido and performance and that can be purchased over the counter at your local health food store or vitamin outlet.

The variety of factors both psychological and physiological that may have adverse effects on our libido and our sexual performance include—but are not limited to—energy levels, circulation, physical fitness, stress, and relationship difficulties with a sexual partner. If any of these factors, or a combination of them, are out of balance, a decreased libido may occur. Through proper diet and a nutritional supplementation program supported by an exercise regime, many of these problems can be eliminated and a positive difference will take place in most situations.

Of course, emotional and psychological issues associated with sexuality can have an impact on the effect of the support program. If an individual is angry at his or her partner, he or she is less likely to experience sexual desire regardless of the appropriate dietary, nutritional, or exercise support. At the same time, a positive attitude about the use of a complete support program often leads to enhanced libido and sexual performance.

Some of the nutritional support factors listed below will help both male and female sexual partners. I don't want you to think that every one of these qualify as "Love Potion #9." I do believe, however, that some of these taken in the right combinations and dosage will spice up your sex drive, sexual performance, and overall health program.

HUMAN GROWTH HORMONE AND SEXUALITY

First, a short class in Hormones 101. I think it will help you to understand the functions and roles of various glands and hormones in your body and will also help you make informed choices about what level of hormone treatment or supplementation you may choose to implement in your life.

The minute you start talking about the human libido you are entering into the complex interconnected hormonal secretion system in the body known as the *endocrine system*. A hormone is a chemical that is produced by an organ or by cells from an organ that directly regulates the activity and output of an organ. In the body, hormones affect everything from muscle growth, to energy level, to the actual function of your organs.

Your endocrine system, which is basically composed of the hypothalamus, pituitary gland, adrenal gland, the pancreas, the thyroid, and the testes or ovaries, is the physical structure that regulates your body clock. Your hypothalamus, which is the starting point of your endocrine system, is where decisions like "This body is 50, its time to reduce hormones by 50 percent" are made.

The body clock is the focal point of any serious antiaging program. Once we understand how it works, we can truly make real progress in first stopping, and then reversing this hormonal version of your Timex. Sexuality, on the hormonal level, really starts in the hypothalamus. It feeds hormones to the pituitary gland. In turn, the pituitary gland sends a luteinizing hormone to the testes or ovaries. The testes create testosterone and the ovaries create estradiol, which flow back to the pituitary gland and the hypothalamus. There, a gonadatropic-releasing hormone is created that sends out signals to the rest of the body. This is what we call *libido*. Now, you are ready to make love.

Just how ready you are depends on the level of hormonal secretion your hypothalamus has determined ought to be released for a person your age. For those of us committed to the Forever Young lifestyle, this is where the fun and the intervention begin.

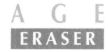

HGH INJECTIONS

Today, physicians are using growth-hormone injections to promote dramatic antiaging effects in people from their mid-30s to their late 80s. It has been well documented that growth-hormone shots are effective in slowing down the aging process. Based on the increasing body of evidence that human-growth-hormone deficiency is exhibited in many adults beginning from age 25 and on, many countries have approved the use of these hGH injections (somatotropin) as a replacement therapy in deficient adults.

The results and efficacy of hGH therapy are strikingly consistent. Those patients that go untreated and have hGH deficiencies are shown to have increased cardiovascular mortality, reduced skeletal muscle strength, reduced exercise capacity, reduced renal plasma flow, defective thermal-regulation and sweat secretion, reduced energy expenditure and basal-metabolic rate, reduced myocardial function, clinical signs of premature arteriosclerosis, and abnormal thyroid metabolism.

hGH-deficient adults also show signs of decreased lean body mass, increased fat body mass, visceral obesity, reduced bone-mineral content, and reduced extra-cellular fluid volume. Other independent groups have reported repaired physiological well-being and somatotropin deficiency as distinct clinical consequences, all of which can be totally eliminated with hGH replacement therapy.

One of the most obvious negative effects of declining hGH levels is an impaired sexual vigor as men and women age. Whether through injections or other methods and programs, the rewards for increasing hGH levels are plentiful and dramatic.

In Chapter Eleven we'll cover, in great depth, how you can implement a complete program to elevate hGH. There we'll thoroughly review its effect, not just on sexuality, but on your overall well-being and good health. We'll give you a complete explanation of how to implement various hGH-elevating alternatives.

DHEA

The good news: DHEA (short for dehydroepiandrosterone) is a hormone produced naturally in the body's endocrine system that provides energy, vitality, sexuality, radiance, muscle growth, disease protection, and a host of other attributes related to positive life forces in the body.

The bad news: As we age, DHEA is the fastest nose-diving hormone in the body. There is, in fact, a dramatic decrease in the production of DHEA. By our mid-40s we are producing less than 50 percent of the levels of our mid-30s. By the time men and women reach their 70s they are producing only 15 percent. Some scientists believe that DHEA is so fundamental to the aging function that its level in your body is considered a biomarker, or an actual measure of your physiological age.

Is this fact important to your sex life? You bet it is. DHEA, which is made from pregnenolone (another key hormone in the body), is converted directly to testosterone and estrogen. Now, if you've dropped 50 percent in DHEA production since your last high school reunion, you can see how your sexual drive and performance could be seriously diminished by the time your next one comes around. A decline in libido often accompanies a decline in DHEA in both women and men.

This was clearly demonstrated in the groundbreaking Massachusetts Male Aging Study, which investigated, among other things, sexual function and activity in men ages 40 to 70. The study not only found that the risk of severe or total impotence increased threefold with age, but that of the 17 hormones measured in each of the men, only one showed a direct and consistent correlation with impotence—and that was DHEA. As DHEA levels declined, the incidence of impotence increased. Fortunately, many men are reporting that DHEA supplementation has renewed their interest in sex and improved their sex lives.

PREGNENOLONE

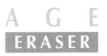

Pregnenolone is made in the body from cholesterol. It is a precursor to DHEA and ultimately may provide many of the same benefits. Pregnenolone is the parent steroid from which all other steroids arise. Consequently, supplementation may provide the necessary precursors for the production of testosterone and other steroids associated with libido.

In one study, the major pathway of pregnenolone metabolism was found to be androgen synthesis, where the formation of DHEA, androstenedione, testosterone, and at least three sulfated androgens takes place. Most people reported "feeling better" after pregnenolone supplementation. Studies demonstrate that pregnenolone enhances our ability to perform on the job while heightening our feelings of well-being. These reported benefits are directly related to increases in sexual desire and performance.

L-ARGININE

Arginine is an essential amino acid. It is one of the eight essential amino acids that your body cannot manufacture from the twenty-two nonessential amino acids in your body. Arginine is one of the leading pro-sexual nutrients that has been shown to contribute to sexual arousal, stamina, and eventual sexual pleasure. Arginine is joined by other amino acids, ornithine, DL-phenylalanine, and tyrosine in its efforts. Arginine may be consumed in foods (nuts, chicken, turkey, and dairy products) or may be taken in food supplement tablets or capsules.

Arginine was always recognized as a limited potential building block. It is now accepted as a great molecule builder and provider of nitrogenous compounds that are the keys to sexual arousal. Durk Pearson and Sandy Shaw did volumes of research showing that L-arginine, taken in large dosages, acts to release growth hormone from the pituitary gland.

YOHIMBINE

Yohimbine is an active alkaloid in a yohimbe bark. For centuries, it has been reported to have aphrodisiac properties. In its synthetic form, yohimbine is the only FDA-approved drug legally considered to be an aphrodisiac and has been used in a number of studies to treat sexual difficulties resulting from a variety of causes.

Yohimbine's aphrodisiac properties benefit both men and women and seem to be a result of two physiological functions. One function is its ability to cause a dilation of the blood vessels, particularly in the genital region. Thus, an increased flow of blood to the penis or vagina may result in improved stimulation. One word of caution: yohimbine may also act as an agent in lowering blood pressure. Those who know they have low blood pressure should, of course, consult their physician and exercise caution using this herb.

The second function of yohimbine is its ability to block presynaptic alpha-2 adrenergic receptors. This blockage results in an increase in parasympathetic cholinergic activity and a decrease in sympathetic adrenergic activity. This is important, since male sexual performance (arousal) is linked to cholinergic activity and to alpha-2 adrenergic blockage.

Viagra and drugs like it do not enhance the libido or cause sexual arousal. These drugs will not work unless and until a man (and if studies prove effective, a woman) is aroused. Yohimbine actually works on the parasympathetic nerve system, and stimulates individuals to feel sexual arousal and sexual urgency. In simpler terms, yohimbine causes an elevation of libido stimulation, and tells the body, "I am interested in making love." The drug Viagra works physically as a vasodilator and tells the body, "I am able to make love."

AVENA SATIVA

Avena sativa has a sedative effect upon the central nervous system. This effect may help to eliminate or reduce any agitation or anxiety that makes sexual performance difficult. Of equal or greater significance is that avena sativa has been demonstrated to free up testosterone, which becomes increasingly bound to various compounds in the body with advancing age. Bound testosterone is not nearly as effective as free testosterone in stimulating the sex drive that leads individuals to engage in sexual activity.

Avena sativa has also been shown to stimulate the release of luteinizing hormone. This is significant because luteinizing hormone is involved in effecting the secretion of certain sexual hormones in women (such as progesterone) as well as in men (testosterone). Women who suffer from dryness of the vaginal tissues may find relief with this herb as it has been proven to facilitate vaginal lubrication.

In 1986, the Institute of Advanced Study of Human Sexuality conducted a study to explore the aphrodisiac effect of avena sativa. Subjects were given 300 mg of avena sativa extract three days a week for six weeks. The subjects were all volunteers and expressed an interest in improving their sexual response and/or partner interaction. Their dysfunction or dissatisfaction ranged from male impotence and female lack of desire or inability to respond sexually, to an interest in making an adequate sex life better.

Both men and women reported enhanced sexual desire, performance, and sensation while taking avena sativa. Men and women were

14 percent more aware of the sexual potential of daily events and of triggered sexual thoughts. Men and women both experienced increased genital sensation accompanying sexual thoughts. The women who completed the study reported a 21 percent increase in lubrication in response to sexual thoughts and fantasies, which resulted in a 19 percent increase in some form of sexual gratification.

MUIRA PUAMA

In Brazil, muira puama has long been valued as an aphrodisiac and tonic for the nervous system. More recent research has validated this botanical's traditional use. At the Institute of Sexology in Paris, a clinical study with 262 patients complaining of lack of sexual desire and/or the inability to attain or maintain an erection was conducted using muira puama. Dr. Jacques Wainburg, one of the world's foremost authorities on sexual function, supervised the study. Within two weeks, 62 percent of males and females diagnosed with loss of libido reported that the treatment had dynamic effects. Over 50 percent of the men treated reported that the treatment was a success with "erection failures."

TRIBULUS TERRESTRIS

Another herb, tribulus terrestris, has been used in treating genital and urinary problems and has been prescribed for treating impotence as a general tonic for centuries. Ayurveda preparation containing tribulus terrestris was used to treat 50 patients complaining of lethargic fatigue and lack of interest in day-to-day activity. The results showed an overall improvement of 45 percent in symptoms.

Of greater significance are studies where the standardized extracts of tribulus terrestris were found to have a stimulating effect on the libido of both men and women. A word of caution: some women experienced a high increase in testosterone levels. Tests of healthy men demonstrated that a five-day treatment of three tablets of the standardized extract of 50 mg or better per day increased levels of testosterone approximately 30 percent.

In another study, a group of men suffering from a range of reproductive disorders (impotence, hypogonadism, infertility) were treated with the standardized extract of the tribulus terrestris. The results confirmed previous positive findings by increasing testosterone levels and improving libido in subjects, with no reported negative side effects.

PRECURSORS TO PERFORMANCE

Of course, no discussion about sex-enhancing drugs would be complete without mention of the most famous of all—Viagra. Viagra has been tremendously successful and has made a lot of men and their partners very happy. Women are currently testing it for use. It is an extremely effective vasodilator, helping blood to flow to the important parts of the body required for sexual performance. But it is not a libido enhancer. There must be libido stimulation for Viagra to work properly. Without a libido boost, it may fail. Unfortunately, if men feel it doesn't work for them, after all of the hype and publicity, they may begin to believe that something is desperately wrong with them. This fear and depression can diminish the libido even more.

I believe that for most people, it is also important to look beyond the previously mentioned nutrients and formulas that have specific sexual-performance properties. It is critical to remember that *overall* health and mental attitude are the real keys to a healthy sex life. When speaking of sexual vigor and vitality, you must take into consideration all of the other items that you may be consuming. Are you taking any antianxiety drugs or hypertension drugs? Any of these may be interfering with your libido, and only a trained physician can tell you what is safe and proper to use to counteract the negative aspects of otherwise positive drugs.

Your ability to be a sexual partner doesn't just happen in one particular zone of the body. I believe that the largest sexual organ in your body is your mind, and the proper mindset is essential to a thriving sex life. We shouldn't underestimate the power of the feelings associated with phrases like, "I'm just not in the mood tonight, honey." Which is why mood elevators should be considered for many people.

The most common mood supporters are St. John's Wort, glutamine peptides, and tonic herbs. Maca is an herb from Peru believed to be a powerful mood enhancer. Catawba is considered the Brazilian aphrodisiac herb because of its mood-elevating properties. Jojoba is a natural tonic. Many people have discovered that jojoba tea helps them feel strong and vigorous—it acts as a natural source of overall good health.

DL-phenylalanine is a powerful mood elevator. We need endorphins to flow through the body, and DL-phenylalanine is a great asset to this because it helps elevate endorphins in the brain at the neurotransmitter level. It can create a feeling of well-being and help put you in a positive state of mind, desiring to participate in sex. Of course, without desire, all of the Viagra in the world, or any other vasodilator, will not work.

Other nutrients critical to good overall health have special significance to your sexuality. Vitamin E, for example, increases the oxygen and blood flow throughout the body, not only from the brain but everywhere else. Another powerful vitamin with sexual benefits is zinc. It is very important to the overall health of your sexual organs. Zinc concentrations are highest in the prostate. Zinc ions actually inhibit the androgen metabolism that can cause prostate problems.

Some women lament, when they reach menopause and post-menopausal years where estrogen levels may decline dramatically, "I've lost it all and I can't do anything about it." But they are wrong. There are phytoestrogens that can reverse the course. Botanicals such as black cohosh, soy germ, chaste tree berry and dong quai can stimulate hormone secretion and have very positive effects. With the right support programs, women in their postmenopausal years can remain sexually active and sometimes even more fulfilling.

Men face another type of problem as they age. Cancer is obviously the most serious of the problems that can occur. The most common prostate problem is enlargement, and make no mistake, prostate problems will definitely affect a man's libido and sex life. One nutrient that is a major contributor to a healthy prostate is saw palmetto, which is very effective in acting directly on the enlarged prostate to reduce the inflammation and pain experienced by many men. Many clinical trials have shown that saw palmetto berries are useful in reducing the inflammation of the prostate in cases of benign prostate hypertrophy (BPH). In fact, saw palmetto extract is so effective at treating BPH that it has been compared to the prescription drug Proscar. During the course of three studies involving 350 men, saw palmetto extract was associated with a significant increase in urinary flow rate and a 50 percent decrease in residual urine volume.

Another important nutrient for prostate health is pygeum. It possesses anti-inflammatory properties that are particularly effective for the prostate. This herb works by inhibiting the formation of the prostaglandins PGE2 and PGF2, well-known mediators of the inflammatory process. Pygeum extract has also been used in the treatment of BPH.

Other common natural ingredients have been shown to aid in promoting a healthy prostate. Cranberry juice powder, for example, works because its acids tend to destroy bacteria present in the urinary tract. Pumpkin seed oil concentrates and the amino acid glycine have been clinically demonstrated to reduce prostate enlargement.

CONCLUSION

Your sex life, in many ways, is a microcosm of your overall health. A healthy sex life relies on a complex interwoven combination of mental attitude, physiological conditioning, and emotional influences. The starting point for reshaping your sexual life and truly renewing a more youthful vitality is discarding the idea that sexual decline must accompany aging. Once you have rebuffed this concept and replaced it with possibility and positive energy and a planned course of intervention, you're on your way to creating a more fulfilling sexual life, no matter what your age.

And last but not least, I believe that to truly love the person you are with may be the most important element in a younger, more meaningful sex life. Don't just chase indiscriminate sexual encounters. Enjoy a healthy, active, and safe love life with the one most important person in your world.

eleven
the forever young
hormones

WITH DR. DAVID LEONARDI

The views expressed in this chapter are strictly those of Dr. David Leonardi as a result of his research through the Cenegenics Clinic. Dr. Leonardi's opinions do not represent the views of the entire hormone replacement therapy medical field. Many physicians in this field differ with some of the opinions expressed by Dr. Leonardi. Hormone replacement therapy can be a vital contribution to any proper age management program. Before starting any program, speak with your personal physician and together seek out whatever authority you choose to utilize in the creation of your own hormone replacement program.

When I was preparing to write this book, I had many moments of anxiety over just what the most important age eraser might be. I honestly could not come to a decision. There is one thing, however, of which I am certain. The hormone system of men and women plays an unparalleled role in determining just how vibrant and energetic their life will be. Oh, we will all age, at least chronologically, but the degree of biological aging will vary greatly from one individual to another. I finally decided that this subject matter had to be put into the hands of someone who lives and works in the arena of hormone therapy every day of his life.

Like Dr. L. Cass Terry, who collaborated with me on the chapter about memory and a healthy brain, Dr. David Leonardi is an expert in antiaging medicine and hormone therapy. He is the medical director of Cenegenics Medical Institute in Las Vegas, Nevada. He has examined me on several occasions, and his observations are included in this book.

I want you to have the latest information on hormonal treatments, and Dr. Leonardi is in the best position to provide the technical answers I feel are needed on this topic.

I've personally had a three-and-a-half-year relationship with the Cenegenics Medical Institute. I have never been on their payroll or received any earnings from them. I make the following observation from the heart: The CEO of Cenegenics is Dr. Alan Mintz, a man who, along with his president and chief financial officer, John Adams, has personally invested a great portion of their life's earnings to get Cenegenics off the ground. Their devotion and passion for what they do far exceed any financial motives.

Over the past three years, Cenegenics Medical Institute has received an enormous amount of press and television coverage. Some of it has been good and some of it not-so-good. The not-so-good comes, I believe, from the sheer desire among certain media to create controversy and sell their "news." What Cenegenics is doing is cutting-edge. They are willing to take the chance of being second-guessed and criticized because they know the truth. And that truth is that if we are ever going to learn to be Forever Young, we must push the envelope with safe, scientific methods supported by data and case histories of people who believe that *aging is not an inevitable occurrence, but a preventable disease.*

I personally can think of no finer hands to put my remaining years into than the totally committed and ethically motivated staff of Cenegenics Medical Institute. Because I believe this, you will find the address and contact information for Dr. David Leonardi, Dr. Alan Mintz, John Adams, and the Cenegenics team in the reference section at the back of this book.

Dr. Leonardi's practice at Cenegenics Medical Institute covers all aspects of slowing the aging process and reversing its symptoms. For this chapter I asked David to only address hormone therapy. He has generously provided me with all of the information that follows. Again, as in Dr. Cass Terry's chapter on the healthy brain, in this chapter I am only the messenger. Dr. Leonardi is the expert who provided me with the information! He has given me a lot of somewhat complex information and supported it with relevant studies. This is such important age-management information that I hope you will read it slowly, and maybe more than once. If you do, I promise you'll learn a great deal!

In this chapter we're going to focus on the hormones that decline as we age, the resulting consequences, and the expectations you may have by regulating their levels. In men, levels of testosterone decline on average 30 percent from age 30 to 50. DHEA and growth hormone decline at similar rates. In women, estradiol, progesterone, and testosterone decrease abruptly with menopause. By the age of 35, many men and women have the melatonin levels of an 80-year-old. Low thyroid syndrome, which can affect men or women, sometimes occurs in this age bracket as well. These are hormones that collectively contributed to the energy, strength, stamina, larger muscle mass, lower body fat, greater libido, and the more "optimistic" outlook of our youth.

HUMAN GROWTH HORMONE (HGH)

Otherwise known as hGH, or *somatotropin*, growth hormone is a polypeptide (protein) hormone synthesized and secreted by the anterior pituitary gland. While in children, especially adolescents, it is secreted throughout the day and night, in adults its release is limited almost exclusively to nighttime. hGH is secreted in short "bursts" that occur with no specific pattern but are associated with stage 3 and 4 sleep, a very deep sleep state. The sleep-related hGH release is believed responsible for the decline in hGH levels as we age. When stage 3 sleep was artificially induced in older men, hGH levels rose dramatically.

After being released into the bloodstream, hGH is quickly metabolized and only lasts about 30 minutes in the bloodstream. While there, however, it manages to get to the liver and induce the liver to make another hormone called IGF-1, or insulin-like growth factor 1. It is IGF-1 that travels through the tissues in our bodies to cause most of the effects that we attribute to hGH. So although IGF-1 is the true effector of the results, *we can only make IGF-1 from the stimulation provided by hGH.*

Modern clinical trials on hGH in adult males were pioneered by Dr. Daniel Rudman, who published his landmark study in *The New England Journal of Medicine* on July 7, 1990. Dr. Rudman supplemented injections of hGH in older men for six months. In this study, he reported an average increase in muscle mass of 8.8 percent. Body fat decreased by over 14 percent, skin thickness increased by 7.1 percent, and bone density in the lumbar spine increased by 1.6 percent. (We now know that more significant changes in bone mass from hormonal therapies take longer than the six months used in Dr. Rudman's study.)

Dr. Rudman's work opened up a new era in society's view of

aging. Aging no longer appeared to be an unavoidable process. No longer did people feel hopeless about the prospects of aging. A whole new era of research opened up to study aging as a treatable disease rather than an inevitable life process. If the release of hGH declines with age and if modulating (adjusting the levels) it offers such terrific results, were the other life-enhancing hormones suffering a similar decline? And, if so, would modulating these other hormones produce similar positive results?

The revolution had begun and now hundreds of thousands around the globe are investigating and participating in hormone modulation. The National Institute on Aging (NIA) just completed a study modeled after Dr. Rudman's to attempt to either verify or refute his findings. The study provided a more in-depth measurement of various outcomes. Other hormones were studied both independently of, and along with, growth hormone. The results of hGH alone, however, were remarkably similar to Dr. Rudman's, lending great credence to his findings and further advancing interest in this exciting field of medicine.

What Can We Expect from Taking hGH?

The list of benefits that have been published from clinical trials are as follows:

➤ Decrease in body fat
➤ Increase in lean body mass (muscle)
➤ Thickening and decreased wrinkling of the skin
➤ Faster wound healing, be it a surgical wound or an injury
➤ Decrease in LDL (bad) cholesterol
➤ Better immune function
➤ Increase in aerobic capacity as a result of increased muscle mass
➤ Less potential risk of being sick or hospitalized
➤ Strengthened immunity
➤ Decrease in diastolic blood pressure
➤ Decrease in the waist-to-hip ratio (meaning body fat is removed preferentially from the waist area where it is associated with a greater risk of heart disease)
➤ Increase in blood flow to the kidneys for the filtering and excretion of waste
➤ Greater feeling of well-being (elevation in mood)

Individuals taking hGH report that their energy level is boosted, that they require less sleep and yet are sleeping much better. They awake more refreshed with a better outlook on life. They don't fatigue as quickly. They handle adversity with greater ease and confidence. Many (not all) have reduced body fat and changed clothing size. They get sick less. They are more motivated to exercise, and workouts are stronger and more enjoyable. Athletic performance has improved. Almost across the board they report thicker, more youthful-appearing skin. They often report functioning more effectively in their business. Some note improvement in memory. A few men have claimed regrowth of scalp hair. Other individuals have noted a reduction in spider veins.

Whether or not hGH will reduce mortality or extend our life span won't be known for several decades. What we do know is that among individuals taking hGH therapy, most experience a substantial enhancement of their quality of life.

Are There Any Risks to Using hGH?

There are no proven risks to using hGH. That is to say, no studies to date have proven that hGH supplementation has ever caused any disease. As with many issues in medicine, there is conflicting data. There is one study that points to a possible association between higher levels of IGF-1 and risk of cancer of the prostate. There are three studies showing that men with prostate cancer had no higher levels of IGF-1 than men of the same age that did not have cancer. There is one study illustrating a possible association between higher IGF-1 and breast cancer in women who had not yet undergone menopause. In this same study, the same thing was not true in breast cancer patients *after* menopause. Yet another study showed that even before menopause there was no difference in IGF-1 levels between a group of women with breast cancer and an age-matched group without breast cancer.

We can come up with many theories about how these variations occur, but any conclusions drawn would be guesses because we simply don't have enough data available to draw a reliable conclusion. This is common because medicine is not an exact science. Human physiology is so complex that there are always a large number of variables that can affect an outcome. To try to isolate one variable among so many parts is difficult at best and often requires a complex statistical analysis that opens the door for even more error. Then there is the issue of bias on the part of the person(s) conducting the study. Before drawing conclusions, physicians like to see a number of studies done with different populations, by different investigators showing similar results, as in the case of studies about estrogen replacement after menopause.

Are There Any Side Effects from hGH?

There are potential side effects from hGH that are relative to the dose. This means that side effects can almost always be avoided by using a conservative dose. In a very sensitive individual who experiences side effects even at a low dose, they are easily alleviated by withdrawing treatment for a week and resuming at an even lower dose. The side effects are related to salt and water retention because hGH can cause sodium to be reabsorbed by the kidneys, decreasing their excretion. This can cause fluid accumulation in the lower legs or around joints and can result in some joint stiffness or aching. This will often be felt in the fingers or another joint where there may be preexisting arthritis. The effect is generally mild and easily controlled with a smaller dose.

How Is hGH Administered?

Growth hormone itself can be administered only by injection. A tiny (30-gauge, 3/8-inch) needle is used and is usually not even felt when it penetrates the skin. This is the same needle diabetics use to inject insulin day in and day out. hGH cannot be taken orally as it is a polypeptide (protein), and instead of absorbing the intact hGH molecule, we would digest it and absorb the resulting amino acids (no different from chicken). Injections are best taken six days a week, once daily, usually in the morning.

The six-day-per-week schedule is based on the theory that one day off each week will keep the pituitary gland more active. All hormones are controlled by a mechanism called "negative feedback." This means that when the amount of hormone in the blood reaches a certain level, it inhibits the gland that produced it from secreting any more. When the hormone is used up and the level drops, secretion resumes. By taking daily injections of hGH it's been theorized (not proven) that we can keep our pituitary shut off and cause it to atrophy to the point where it might no longer produce. Taking off one day per week is designed therefore to "exercise" our pituitary glands.

Morning injections are preferred since our own hGH is secreted during sleep. Bedtime injections are almost certain to exert a negative feedback, decreasing our own production of the hormone. By 5:00 A.M. the pituitary has completed its secretion of hGH, for the most part, at least until the next evening. If we inject in the morning, that dose is metabolized by the time our pituitary gears up again, avoiding any negative feedback.

Some individuals seem to get better results dividing the daily dose into two injections, one in the morning and one in the evening. Although this appears contradictory to the negative feedback theory, physicians use blood levels to determine the optimal dose for each individual. The degree of negative feedback can vary substantially among users. When doctors prescribe two doses daily, they also have the patient inject the majority of the dose in the morning, keeping the evening dose on the low side to minimize any possible negative feedback.

Because hGH is administered by subcutaneous injection, some researchers believe its impact in oxidizing fat is greater locally at the injection site than anywhere else, it can be useful in "spot reducing." Most men therefore will inject around the waist and women seem to prefer tummy or hip injections. The injection site should vary somewhat to avoid dimpling from fat loss in one location. Not all researchers agree that this effect has been sufficiently substantiated.

What's the Cost of hGH Therapy?

hGH therapy is not cheap! Programs starts at about $600 a month partly because of the expensive manufacturing practice of recombinant DNA technology, and partly because current patent protection keeps price support high. Patents may expire in 2003 if applications for extension are denied, and prices may come down.

Is hGH for You?

Although most people do, not everyone feels better on hGH. Most doctors advise committing to a three-month trial to see how an individual will feel and perform. If the benefits don't appear, there's no harm in stopping the therapy. In the opinion of Dr. Leonardi (and it is an opinion I share) the potential advantages are far too great to not at least give it a try if it is a financial possibility for you. A physician trained and experienced in antiaging medicine can help you make the decision.

There may be other hormones and/or treatments that would benefit you more or that would be best used in conjunction with hGH. There is no substitute for a complete evaluation by a qualified antiaging physician with a global approach. You should find an antiaging specialist who considers not only hGH, but other hormones as well as nutrition, exercise, avoidance of environmental toxins, stress reduction, and all the other aspects of preventive health that are available to us today.

SEX HORMONES—NOT JUST FOR SEX

I present the following information on pregnenolone and DHEA with the studies that support the theory. However, there are those who believe that more data are necessary to substantiate the information. I believe you should have the chance to form your own decision.

There are nine important hormones in this category. One, pregnenolone, is actually a sex hormone precursor that is made in the adrenal gland from cholesterol. The other eight (four male and four female) are synthesized from pregnenolone.

Pregnenolone itself has no influence on sexual function. It is classified as a *neuroactive* steroid. That means it exerts an effect on nerve cells, particularly in the brain. In laboratory rats and mice, very high doses of pregnenolone injected directly into the brain have been shown to improve memory and enhance learning. There are no *human* studies published on the effects of an oral dose of pregnenolone on memory. The closest we've come to that is in a study showing that a large intravenous injection of pregnenolone in rats did improve learning. Pound for pound, this was equivalent to a 4.3-gram dose in a 154-pound human (a huge dose).

The association between pregnenolone and mood is worth noting. Pregnenolone levels in spinal fluid (the fluid that bathes our brain) were found to be substantially lower in depressed than nondepressed patients. Furthermore, if the depressed person was having a bad day, the pregnenolone level was even lower!

So you might think pregnenolone would be a mood elevator. The problem is, no one knows just what happens to an oral dose of pregnenolone once we swallow it. Is it well absorbed from the intestine into the bloodstream? Does it cross the blood-brain barrier, that membrane between the blood and the brain that selectively screens compounds in the blood to allow only certain ones in? If so, once in the brain, does it turn on or off the correct receptor, in the correct area, to stimulate improvement of memory or elevation of mood in humans? No one knows the answers to these questions because the clinical studies have not been done. As a naturally occurring substance, pregnenolone cannot be patented. So no one has been willing to spend the large amount of money required to study and publish results.

Maybe a graduate student will someday be interested enough to obtain a government grant to do a human clinical trial with pregnenolone. Until then, we must decide whether or not to use it from the small amount of indirect information we already have. I personally do take pregnenolone because I believe it to be harmless and for the chance that it might help preserve my memory. Should you decide to try pregnenolone, most physicians recommend being conservative and staying between 20 and 100 mg per day.

The most important male hormones are DHEA, androstenedione, testosterone, and dihydrotestosterone. On the female side are progesterone, estriol, estradiol, and estrone. Keep in mind that the labels *male* and *female* only designate the gender in which a particular hormone is dominant. *This does not mean that the hormone is not found in the opposite sex.* In fact, all four of the male hormones can be measured in women, and the female hormones can be measured in men. Some actually play extremely important roles in the opposite sex.

DHEA

DHEA (dehydroepiandrosterone) is a male sex hormone (androgen), yet is a critical player in the health and well-being of women. Like pregnenolone, it is made in the adrenal glands. Although it is the weakest of the androgens, it has other benefits that are more important than its androgenic effect. It has been shown to be a potent stimulator of immunity by increasing the activity of a very important lymphocyte in the control of infections and cancer. DHEA has also been proven to be a critical component in the process of antibody production.

DHEA and Depression

DHEA has been related to mood as well. Dr. Barrett-Conner and associates from the University of California, San Diego, studied seven hormones in women for evidence of their effect on mood. Of the seven, only DHEA sulfate (DHEAS) levels were consistently found to be lower in depressed than nondepressed patients. DHEAS is made from DHEA in our bodies very shortly after an oral dose of DHEA.

When women reach menopause, the brain loses its ability to respond to endorphins, the neurotransmitters that provide a wonderful feeling of well-being. A study by Stomati and colleagues from Italy showed that supplementing DHEA restored the responsiveness of the endorphin receptor to its premenopausal level. Another study by Wolkowitz and colleagues at the University of California, San Francisco, showed DHEA to decrease symptoms by over 50 percent in 5 of 11 patients classified with major depression.

DHEA and Body Composition

When women take DHEA, their bodies generally convert some of it into testosterone, a much stronger male hormone. Testosterone levels in most women therefore, rise substantially. Although there are studies that show no increase in muscle mass or strength in women on DHEA, most women seem to enjoy a feeling of greater strength, energy, and libido when taking DHEA. Maybe the studies were too short-term to demonstrate this response and perhaps results would've been better if the women had been on an exercise program. Certainly more studies are needed to clarify the effects of DHEA on body composition in women. In men, DHEA has been shown, in two out of three studies, to decrease body fat and increase muscle mass.

Premenopausal (menstruating) women should be careful with DHEA because it can alter estrogen levels and cause menstrual irregularity. As with all the hormones, whether available by prescription or over the counter, DHEA should only be used under the supervision of a physician trained in hormone modulation and with follow-up blood or salivary levels to avoid side effects and complications.

Too much DHEA in women can lead to acne and/or growth of facial hair (hirsuitism). Another consideration in women taking DHEA is that as testosterone levels rise they could experience a decrease in the good cholesterol, HDL. Lower HDL levels can increase risk of heart disease. A physician well trained in hormone modulation will know how to screen for and alleviate this problem. This is just one more reason to seek professional monitoring for your hormone program.

Ironically, in men DHEA taken as a supplement is not converted by the body to testosterone. It is converted to the female hormone estrone!

So men too should be careful of the dose taken to avoid feminizing symptoms from high levels of estrogens. Finding the right dose for you is the key to enjoying the benefits without side effects. A typical dose of DHEA is 25 mg one to three times a day for women or men.

A G E
ERASER

TESTOSTERONE

Testosterone is the quintessential male hormone. In men, it is made in the testicle from its precursor, androstenedione. Remember, however, that in the study published in *The Journal of the American Medical Association* in 1999, oral androstenedione given to men did not lead to increased production of testosterone. Hormones are handled differently in the body depending on their source.

Testosterone truly contributes to our ability to increase lean body mass (muscle). It also helps to trim body fat, although not as efficiently as hGH. Testosterone levels in men decline by about 1 percent per year between the ages of 30 and 50. At the same time, the protein in the blood that binds testosterone, partly decreasing its activity, is on the rise. The result is a substantial drop in the free (unbound) testosterone available to stimulate testosterone receptors.

In women, testosterone declines abruptly at menopause just like estrogen and progesterone, although it is often overlooked by many doctors who are unaware of its importance in women. Testosterone receptors are found throughout the body in virtually every organ and tissue including the brain, heart, skeletal muscle, fat, penis, and clitoris. Can there be any mystery as to why a 50-year-old doesn't perform like a 30-year-old?

One of the best research projects to date on the use of testosterone in aging men is seen in the work of Drs. Mark Blackman and Mitch Harmon in a study conducted by the National Institute on Aging between 1995 and 1999. Although results have not been published at the time of this writing, much has been reported by the researchers at various medical conferences.

The research project was a double-blind placebo-controlled trial in men aged 62 to 85. Some men received testosterone alone and others received testosterone plus hGH. Both of these groups were compared to a group taking a placebo. Even though the dose of testosterone supplemented in these men was fairly low (about half of that typically used in clinical practice), the effect on lean body mass and muscle strength was dramatic. Testosterone itself was significantly more effective than placebo or hGH in increasing lean body (muscle) mass *and* strength. It was also effective in reducing body fat, although not as much as hGH. Testosterone use had no effect on blood pressure.

Even more important, there was no increase in prostate-specific antigen (PSA), the universal marker for prostate enlargement and cancer, over the six months of the study in those men on testosterone. Side effects of testosterone in this study were nil. It was extremely well tolerated. Unfortunately, the NIA study did not involve the use of testosterone in women. This would have validated and popularized the tremendous benefit physicians in antiaging medicine are seeing in postmenopausal women who supplement testosterone (or its precursor in women, DHEA). Testosterone's influence spreads far beyond muscle mass and body fat. It is a critical component for optimal function of the brain, heart, and sex organs and in the formation of bone and blood.

Testosterone Is Bliss

Low levels of testosterone have been correlated in good clinical studies with depression. Testosterone replacement is often associated with an increase in emotional uplift and drive, as well as an improved feeling of well-being. There is also the obvious correlation that as men and women age, testosterone levels and cognitive ability decline. The cognitive decline is affected by multiple factors, some of which are yet to be discovered. How much of it is due to testosterone and other hormones is uncertain, but there is evidence of hormonal influence.

A Matter of the Heart

Testosterone is a known dilator of coronary arteries and has been shown to allow patients with coronary artery disease to exercise longer. Testosterone builds muscle by increasing the synthesis of protein in muscle tissue. The heart is a muscle and there are testosterone receptors in the heart. The heart enlarges in a healthy way when we participate in aerobic exercise. It stands to reason that this growth is assisted by testosterone in the same way that it is in skeletal muscle.

The effect of testosterone on cholesterol is more controversial as there are data on both sides of the fence. Medicine is not an exact science. Because there are conflicting data, this is an issue that must be addressed individually with each patient and is the reason we need a physician to monitor therapy. HDL cholesterol often drops in individuals on testosterone. In other patients there is no significant effect. Once discovered, a decline in HDL is usually easily remedied by changes in the diet, a decrease in the dose of testosterone, or the use of an HDL-raising nutrient or medicine. Other things that should be considered in this situation are the levels of the other types of cholesterol, triglycerides, and the overall risk factors for heart disease. A good physician will not make a decision based on only one facet of your health, regardless of its popularity in the media. The variable effect of testosterone is no reason to avoid testosterone and its benefits. It is simply a matter of your doctor monitoring your lipids and managing your situation individually.

Testosterone and Libido

Testosterone is well known to stimulate libido in men. This is very common; but blood levels of testosterone do not always correlate with sex drive. There are men with strong sex drives who have very low levels of testosterone and occasionally men with high levels whose libido is low. Some physicians think this has to do with a man's level of the female hormone estradiol relative to his level of testosterone. Their theory is that high levels of estradiol blunt the effect of testosterone by binding to testosterone receptors or by increasing the level of sex hormone binding globulin (the protein that binds both testosterone and estradiol) enough to bind up more of the testosterone.

Dr. Leonardi tells me that at Cenegenics Medical Institute, physicians control estradiol levels in all male patients by using a small dose of a medication that inhibits estrogen production. By doing this they're able to raise testosterone to the upper limit of normal and still keep estradiol levels well within the normal range. Even so, they still have an occasional patient whose libido doesn't respond. This could be due to a nutritional deficiency or other metabolic problem not yet discovered.

It's extremely important though, that your doctor watches your estradiol level and controls it if you are supplementing testosterone. Fortunately, the vast majority of men who use testosterone respond with an increase in libido. Libido is synonymous with sex drive and is a completely separate issue from erectile function—the ability to achieve and maintain an erection. The studies on the effect of testosterone on erectile dysfunction in men don't show that it helps erectile function; but they have all been short-term studies.

In Dr. Leonardi's practice, a number of men on testosterone have experienced an improvement in erectile function, although it usually takes 8 to 12 months. Once serious causes such as circulatory or neural defects are excluded, testosterone supplementation is clearly the best first approach to erectile dysfunction before moving on to drugs, because if successful, it is treating the true cause of the problem rather than eliminating a symptom. And testosterone therapy also offers many other health benefits.

Testosterone and Bone Density

Bone density is an extremely important issue in health and aging. Loss of bone density makes bones weaker and more brittle, which can result in unnecessary fractures that occur with little or no trauma. What a tragedy when someone who might otherwise live another 25 healthy years dies or becomes incapacitated from surgery for a broken hip when the fracture is due to a preventable disease!

Testosterone is extremely important in building and maintaining bone density. Testosterone administration to men with low levels contributes to a steady increase in bone strength. This is at least partly because some testosterone is converted to estradiol in the body. Estradiol is the most important hormone for bone density in both men and women. This is one reason that when physicians control estradiol levels in men receiving testosterone, they're careful to keep the level from dropping too far. Too much reduction of estradiol in men can lead to accelerated bone loss as well as an increased risk of brain aging, coronary disease, and possibly colon cancer. There are studies that show that quality of life in older men is better with estradiol levels in the higher rather than lower part of the normal range.

Testosterone and Side Effects

Testosterone is well known to stimulate the formation of red blood cells in the bone marrow. Red cells carry oxygen from our lungs to our tissues. The condition of insufficient red cells is termed *anemia* and causes fatigue and weakness. Anemia can also make us more susceptible to a number of other diseases. Supplementing testosterone helps keep up a healthy production of red cells, which in addition to preventing anemia helps improve energy and raise exercise tolerance. A problem can occur, however, with an overproduction of red blood cells in people on testosterone. This is termed *polycythemia,* a condition that increases blood viscosity—thickness. Higher blood viscosity can lead to an increased risk of stroke or heart attack.

Does this mean testosterone should be avoided? Absolutely not! Once again, each person should be treated individually. A red blood cell count should be done every six months and if it is elevated, donate blood. Donating blood periodically is, by the way, one of the healthiest things to do for most men. Not only is it spiritually satisfying but it also helps to lower body iron stores, which increase oxidative stress. For those whose blood cannot be accepted by your blood bank owing to a chronic infection or the use of a particular drug, phlebotomy—the removal of a unit of blood—can be done by your doctor in his office and is covered by most insurance if your red cell count is elevated.

Like hGH, side effects with testosterone are related to the size of the dose and are easily controlled by reducing the dose. They include acne, thinning of scalp hair, new growth of facial hair, and emotional irritability or aggressiveness—which is the source of the term *testy*. There is also the potential for testicular atrophy in men. Again, these are easily controlled by adjusting the dose.

In summary:

➤ Testosterone is extremely important to quality of life in both men and women whose level has declined below the optimal range.
➤ Supplementing testosterone has many benefits as well as potential pitfalls that can be avoided by careful surveillance and management by a qualified antiaging physician.

Monitor Your Dihydrotestosterone

As powerful as testosterone is, there is one hormone on the block that even testosterone fears! Dihydrotestosterone (DHT) is made in our bodies from testosterone. Its androgenic potency is triple that of testosterone.

DHT is found in high concentrations in enlarged prostates and vigorously stimulates growth receptors in the prostate. It also contributes to male pattern baldness. DHT levels can occasionally rise in men who supplement testosterone, particularly if it's administered as a skin cream or gel. It's not felt to be important in women because they use much smaller doses of testosterone and have no prostate. This is just one more item that needs to be watched carefully when you are supplementing testosterone.

Physicians must be careful to keep DHT in the normal range. If it rises above the norm, they simply reduce the dose of testosterone, change the way it's administered, or use an enzyme blocker called *finasteride* (Proscar or Propecia) to control it. Some antiaging doctors feel DHT levels should be allowed to rise and some even administer DHT. Dr. Leonardi doesn't feel the research supports this and doesn't wish to put his patients at risk for prostate disease. If long-term studies someday support the safety of DHT he says he will change his mind, but at this point, he believes that the risk outweighs the benefit.

How Is Testosterone Given?

Testosterone is available by prescription in various forms. There are various transdermal patches. It is Dr. Leonardi's opinion that the patches are short on potency and also expensive. Transdermal creams or gels that are applied once or twice a day are better for potency but very often cause a substantial rise in DHT in men. This is because the enzyme that converts testosterone to DHT is concentrated in hair follicles. Applying testosterone to the skin, therefore, gives the follicles "first right of refusal" to convert it to DHT before it even reaches the blood as testosterone.

Creams or gels are the best way to administer testosterone in women because they don't have to be concerned about DHT. Another method is the implantation of pellets under the skin by a minor surgical procedure. These pellets release testosterone steadily for about six months. They work well as long as the dose is chosen correctly. If the dose is too high, you either live with it for the six months, which can be risky, or the doctor goes digging to retrieve a few pellets. If the dose is too low, then supplementation will be necessary with a cream or injection. I tend to believe this to be the best option for most people.

It is Dr. Leonardi's opinion that injectable testosterone is the most effective and safest route of administration. Blood levels respond well. He reports that his patients are pleased with the effect. DHT tends to remain well controlled without the use of finasteride. Men generally prefer to give themselves a shot in the buttocks once a week to using a cream every day. Patients are taught how to inject themselves in the doctor's office and usually have no problems with incorrect technique, as long as regular blood workups are performed and evaluated.

ESTROGEN REPLACEMENT THERAPY

The term *estrogen* refers to a group of steroid hormones that promote development of the female genital tract in the fetus and the development of female secondary-sex characteristics in young girls. Estrogens stimulate growth of breasts and along with progesterone are primarily responsible for the changes in the uterus that occur during the menstrual cycle. They are also responsible for the normal function and lubrication of the vagina.

Along with progesterone, estrogens are produced by the ovaries, which at menopause undergo involution (atrophy) and cease to produce hormones. At that point there is a huge drop in the level of estrogens. The three primary natural human estrogens are estriol, estradiol, and estrone. Estriol and estrone are relatively weak in their activity compared to estradiol, the strongest of the estrogens.

Premarin is the brand name for a group of conjugated estrogen compounds that are not found naturally in humans and are extracted and purified from the urine of pregnant mares. Premarin, although not a natural human hormone, has many of the same effects on postmenopausal symptoms as the natural ones. Like the natural estrogens, Premarin has been shown to relieve hot flashes and depression, arrest or slow bone loss, decrease risk for cardiovascular disease, and reduce risk for colon cancer and Alzheimer's disease in postmenopausal women. This is an impressive list of benefits, not to mention that taking estrogens postmenopause statistically results in better health and longer life expectancy despite the increased risk for breast cancer seen with their use. This statistical benefit is great. However, it's great *only if your risk for breast cancer is "normal."* If your mother or a sister has had breast cancer, then you are considered to be at higher risk and should discuss this with your physician, weighing the increased risk against the benefits before beginning a course of estrogen replacement.

Natural vs. Synthetic

Many physicians are now promoting the use of natural estrogens over the synthetic or conjugated ones. (Synthetic means made in a laboratory from a test tube. Conjugated estrogens are purified from horse urine so technically they are not synthetic, but nonetheless are not *natural* to humans. So we'll include them in the term *synthetic* for this chapter.)

Dr. Leonardi agrees with the recommendation of natural estrogens, although not because any proof of their benefit has been shown. Many say that the data on the increased risk of breast cancer are because the studies were done using synthetic estrogens. The studies *were* done using synthetics. But so were the studies that showed all the benefits of estrogens. In fact, Wyeth-Ayerst, the manufacturer of Premarin and Prempro, has done such a great job of marketing that almost all subjects in studies on estrogen have been on oral synthetic estrogens.

We don't have research studies comparing natural versus synthetic estrogen and their relative merits versus risks. So if an author is going to suggest that cancer risk is associated only with the synthetics, he's on no firmer ground than those who say all the benefits are available only from synthetics! The truth most likely is that the benefits and risks are very similar, since both result in the same increase in serum or salivary levels of estradiol and that is primarily the way they work.

Now the question is: "Why should you favor natural over synthetic if they appear to be equivalent in benefit and risk?" Well, the first obvious answer is I would much prefer to put a molecule into my body identical to the one made by my own gland than a man-made one designed to be a replacement. There just may be some effect in the synthetic that my body won't like and it may not let me know it until I'm in that tunnel headed for the angel with the bright light!

But there are two other important reasons to use natural human estrogen. It involves the breakdown of estradiol in the body to its downstream by-products. One of these, 16 alpha-hydroxy estrone (16ahe) has been shown to be carcinogenic in test tube, animal, and human studies, and its levels are felt to be a major determinate of breast cancer risk. 16ahe is not a by-product of the other two natural estrogens—estriol and estrone. They appear to carry much less risk and using them may lower your risk of breast cancer. Unfortunately, they are of such low potency that they don't work well alone and so are used along with estradiol in a triple estrogen cream. It stands to reason that using the triple estrogen cream requires lower levels of estradiol than straight estradiol or conjugated estrogens since some effect will be provided by the estriol and estrone components. Lower estradiol should result in less risk since there will be less 16ahe produced.

The second reason is that the natural estrogens are available in a transdermal cream, gel, or patch, and synthetics are available only in tablet (oral) form. This is important because when estrogens are taken orally they are absorbed from the intestine into a specific group of veins that carry them to the liver before going to the rest of the body.

In this "first pass" through the liver, estrogen interferes with the liver's production of IGF-1, the hormone made in response to hGH and that brings about nearly all the beneficial effects of hGH. Oral estrogens decrease by at least 15 percent the level of IGF-1 in the blood.

The fat gain that accompanies estrogen (Premarin, birth control pills, etc.) use is almost certainly due to the decrease in IGF-1. That's not to mention less gain of all the other benefits brought about by IGF-1. When the estrogen is absorbed via the skin it is distributed throughout the body to its receptor sites, and has no effect on IGF-1 production in the liver. This is the reason that none of Dr. Leonardi's patients at Cenegenics receive oral estrogens, synthetic or natural. One of his favorite things is to see his patients lose weight when he takes them off Premarin and puts them on natural estrogen cream.

AGE ERASER

I3C

There is a nutrient in cruciferous vegetables (broccoli, cauliflower, cabbage, brussels sprouts) that greatly decreases the production of 16ahe from estradiol. It is called indole-3-carbinol (I3C). This remarkable nutrient is so effective that one researcher says that it probably reduces the risk of breast cancer in women on estrogen replacement down to the level of those abstaining from estrogen. If this is proven to be the case, women on estrogen can have the best of both worlds—all the benefit with no increase in risk! In addition, there is now evidence that I3C also is effective at preventing cervical cancer. The therapeutic amount of I3C is the amount found in one-third of a cabbage. For those who would like to have the I3C without the cabbage, it is available as a supplement. The therapeutic dose is 300 mg per day. Every one of Dr. Leonardi's female patients takes I3C. It is available at some vitamin shops.

To sum it up:

➤ Estrogen is crucial to the health of postmenopausal women unless you have a first-degree relative with breast cancer.
➤ The natural estrogens are preferable over synthetics for a number of reasons.
➤ Transdermal administration (cream, gel, or patch) is better than oral dosing.
➤ I3C is a must for all women who wish to prevent breast cancer.

PROGESTERONE

Like estrogen, progesterone is a steroid hormone made and secreted by the ovary. Progesterone works together with estrogen to coordinate the female reproductive (menstrual) cycle. While estrogen dominates the first half of the cycle to build up the lining of the uterus, progesterone takes over in the second half to preserve this nutritious lining in case a fertilized egg decides to make its home there.

If pregnancy occurs, progesterone levels remain high to support the uterine lining and the developing fetus. If there is no pregnancy, the progesterone level drops and this triggers a release of the uterine lining and menstrual bleeding. Beyond this, progesterone has a number of other effects on the body more relevant to aging (or better, the inhibition of aging).

The most well-known effect of progesterone in regard to aging is its effect on bone metabolism. Although estrogen has always received most of the credit for preventing postmenopausal osteoporosis, progesterone is now known to play an equally important part. In fact, the combination of the two work as impressively against osteoporosis as they do in regulating the reproductive cycle. The earliest proof of the role of progesterone in the prevention of osteoporosis came from a study published in *The Journal of Clinical Investigation* in May 1986. In it, B. L. Riggs and colleagues showed that substantial lumbar spine bone loss occurs in women in the premenopausal years before estrogen levels have dropped. This is a period of time when progesterone levels in the second part of the cycle begin to gradually decline, with variations from month to month.

Other studies have also linked this decline in progesterone to bone loss in premenopausal women and have shown that supplementing progesterone in the second half of the cycle prevents it. Dr. Leonardi often sees a decline in progesterone levels in women approaching menopause while their menstrual periods remain regular and their estrogen levels remain normal. Although both of these hormones are involved in slowing the rate of osteoporosis, their functions are very different. To understand this you must realize that bone is a very dynamic living tissue. It is constantly tearing down and rebuilding. The teardown is done by cells called *osteoclasts*. The rebuilding is done by *osteoblasts*.

In the development of osteoporosis, the activity of osteoclasts is greater than that of osteoblasts, so we suffer bone loss. This can be due to hormone imbalance, nutritional deficiencies, genetic makeup, or other illness. Well, it just so happens that one of progesterone's jobs is to stimulate osteoblasts, or hasten bone buildup. So as progesterone levels decline in the premenopausal period, an associated decrease in osteoblastic activity causes loss of bone density. Estrogen's job is to slow the action of the osteoclasts, and therefore slow bone breakdown.

Supplementing both hormones after menopause works better than using estrogen alone. Dr. Leonardi frequently starts women on a low dose of natural progesterone when they show a decreased level in the second half of their cycle as they approach menopause. They take progesterone only on cycle days 14 through 25. This not only helps to prevent bone loss but often boosts mood and energy level and reduces anxiety.

Progesterone also affects neurons in the brain. While estrogen has an antidepressant effect and can be slightly stimulating, progesterone has a calming effect. Once again the two hormones work together to balance each other. The exact dose of progesterone used is determined by each woman's levels measured in the blood or saliva. There is great variation, so each woman should be evaluated individually.

Another role of progesterone in the postmenopausal period is the prevention of endometrial cancer. The risk of this disease increases with the use of estrogen after menopause. A number of studies have confirmed that the risk of endometrial cancer in women on both estrogen and progesterone is reduced to the level of those women on no hormone replacement therapy.

There is universal agreement that women who have not had their uterus removed should always be on both hormones after menopause. Controversy arises when a woman has had a hysterectomy. Most traditional physicians ignore the role of progesterone in these women. They think of progesterone only as a protection from endometrial cancer in those women on estrogen who still have their uterus. They are not recognizing the benefits of stimulating bone production and balancing mood. Dr. Leonardi has found progesterone to be effective for women with or without a uterus.

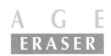

MELATONIN

Melatonin is a hormone synthesized and secreted by the pineal gland in the brain. Its chemical structure is called an *indoleamine*. An indoleamine is an amino acid with an "indole" chemical structure attached to it. In the case of melatonin the amino acid is tryptophan. Since melatonin is well known to induce sleep, L-tryptophan is often used for the same purpose. Melatonin is secreted by the pineal as part of our circadian rhythm, which means that levels are much higher at night and very low in the daytime.

Levels of melatonin peak at around age 13 and decline steeply thereafter. *By the time we are 35, melatonin levels are at the same level as an 80-year-old.* The perception of light by the retina of our eyes triggers the pineal gland to stop releasing melatonin. That's why being sure your room is dark is the first step in treating a sleep disorder.

Sleep disorder is more common in the blind because without the perception of light they lack the circadian cycle of melatonin, so they produce it more steadily around the clock. Melatonin actually regulates our circadian rhythm (daytime/nighttime scheduling of hormone release), which gives it a big influence on many other hormones and functions in our body.

Melatonin's value as a sleeping aid is that as a natural hormone it doesn't influence sleep *architecture*. Now you know I'm not an architect, so what do I mean by sleep architecture? Architecture refers to the structure or the sequence of the stages of sleep we undergo after falling asleep. We begin with the lightest, stage 1 and progress to stage 4 or REM sleep, the deepest and most restful stage. Sleeping pills, alcohol, and tranquilizers, while helping us to fall asleep, alter sleep architecture, so we fail to reach the deeper, more restful stages, resulting in lower-quality sleep.

Jean-Louis and colleagues at the University of California, San Diego, published a study in *The Journal of Pineal Research* in 1998. They gave elderly people 6 mg of melatonin at bedtime in a placebo-controlled trial. While in the melatonin group there was no increase in total sleep, it took them less time to fall asleep and they experienced fewer transitions from sleep to awake. The melatonin group also showed a significant decrease in depressed moods and improvement in memory.

Because melatonin regulates circadian rhythm and aids in sleep, it can be used for jet lag to move the circadian phase forward or backward depending on which direction you're flying. Taking melatonin at bedtime a few days prior to, during, and a few days after a long trip was shown to help a majority of people feel more rested and energetic in a study published in *The Medical Letter*.

Melatonin Is Not Just for Sleep

Melatonin has also been shown to be a powerful cancer fighter as well as an antioxidant. R. J. Reiter and colleagues published a study in the journal *Aging* in 1995. They showed melatonin to be a powerful fighter against free radicals. Although this was an in vitro (test tube) study, they also showed a number of benefits in rats fed melatonin. It blocked free radical damage induced by ionizing radiation and free radical–producing chemicals, preventing damage that would normally occur to the DNA under the same conditions.

Melatonin's anticancer properties were demonstrated by Hill and colleagues of the University of Arizona in their study published in *Cancer Research* in November 1998. Melatonin was added to a tissue culture of breast cancer cells. Adding the melatonin decreased the rate of cell division by 60–78 percent! The amount of melatonin used was equivalent to normal nighttime levels in human plasma.

When the cancer cells exposed to melatonin were examined under an electron microscope, extensive damage to important cell structures was seen. When the cells were removed and placed in a melatonin-free medium, the growth rate returned to normal, proving it was the melatonin and no other factor that inhibited the cancer.

In a study published in *Epidemiology Resources*, Feychting and colleagues found that blind people have 31 percent less overall cancer than sighted people. In the blind, light fails to influence the pineal gland, so melatonin levels are much higher, apparently providing a powerful protective influence against cancer.

Side effects from melatonin, as in other hormones, are easily controlled by adjusting the dose. These effects include morning grogginess and experiencing vivid dreams that may be pleasant or unpleasant. The effective dose varies greatly by individual from 0.5 to 1.5 mg taken orally or sublingually at bedtime. Although physicians can check salivary levels of the hormone, the best method of determining the correct dose is to start low and increase it until you are getting a restful night's sleep. Reduce the dose if you have bothersome dreams or if you're too groggy in the morning. Most people seem to do quite well with 1 mg at bedtime. In a few people, melatonin causes sleeplessness. Those individuals should obviously not take melatonin!

In summary:

➤ Melatonin has antioxidant and anticancer benefits.

- ➤ It is useful as a sleeping aid.
- ➤ It helps alleviate jet lag.
- ➤ It should be taken only at bedtime.
- ➤ The dose should be individualized.

THYROID HORMONE

Thyroid hormone use is one of the most controversial topics in medicine, not only in determining who should be treated but what dose and in which of the several available forms it should be given. Dr. Leonardi feels that there is no doubt that a few people will benefit in a very big way with supplementation of low-dose thyroid hormone even though their blood levels appear "normal." So let's examine what thyroid hormone does. The thyroid's effects are far-reaching: it regulates the body's metabolic rate and energy production. *In doing this it affects virtually every other hormone and system in the body.*

Production of thyroid hormone by the thyroid gland can be normal (euthyroid), too high (hyperthyroid), or too low (hypothyroid). We are only going to talk about the hypothyroid condition. The symptoms of low thyroid are so extensive and common and overlap with so many other diagnoses that anyone who reads the list begins to feel he or she is a victim. But you must be careful with that assumption!

By far the most common symptom in thyroid deficiency is fatigue. Unfortunately, fatigue can be caused by dozens of other problems and low thyroid is most often not the issue. But even when low thyroid is the answer, the thyroid blood test may be normal. Here is where it is important to have a knowledgeable physician who listens. You must always interpret thyroid blood tests in the context of how you feel. The most important and most often measured thyroid hormones are T-3 and T-4.

The thyroid gland makes and secretes both, but most of our T-3 (the stronger of the two) comes from the conversion of T-4 into T-3 in the liver, heart, and kidney. It is also very helpful to measure the pituitary hormone TSH (thyroid stimulating hormone). TSH is the pituitary gland's messenger to stimulate the thyroid gland when it is underactive, causing it to make more thyroid hormone in the way a thermostat controls a heater. When levels of T-3 and T-4 are below adequate, the pituitary is able to sense the problem and respond with higher levels of TSH.

When the thyroid blood test shows an elevated TSH, the diagnosis is easy—hypothyroidism—even if the T-3 and T-4 are normal. Confusion begins when you are tired for no other apparent reason (and remember, there can be many) and your thyroid hormone levels and TSH are normal. This could represent the low T-3 syndrome, a diagnosis originally made to explain low thyroid function in very ill patients in the hospital. These are people who, because they have abnormal metabolism, are slow at converting T-4 into T-3. The result is low or near-low levels of T-3, normal or even high levels of T-4, and because the T-4 hasn't dropped, the TSH is not raised by the pituitary.

Some physicians instruct their patients to take their temperature for several days to help with the diagnosis. If it is consistently low, it may indicate a low thyroid state even with normal blood testing. Dr. Leonardi believes it is important, though, to avoid using temperature as the only indicator of how much thyroid hormone to take. This can lead to overtreatment if the temperature doesn't respond for other reasons or if an error is made in measuring it. It's important to monitor thyroid use by tracking symptoms and correlating them with the blood levels of T-3, T-4, and TSH. Overtreatment with thyroid hormone can cause bone loss leading to osteoporosis. Since antiaging physicians believe in optimal and not just adequate levels of hormones, they are generally more willing to try a patient on low-dose thyroid replacement to see if they improve in the areas of energy, mood, stamina, and/or mental acuity. However, they always have to be aware of blood levels and not overprescribe.

In summary:

> The thyroid's function is far-reaching in its influence.
> If other causes of fatigue have been considered and the thyroid tests are normal, low T-3 syndrome should also be considered.
> Blood tests and reevaluation of symptoms are critical in monitoring the success of a therapeutic trial of low-dose thyroid hormone.
> Measurement of basal body temperature can also be helpful.

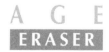

FIND A KNOWLEDGEABLE ANTIAGING PHYSICIAN

Aging is a preventable disease. We simply don't yet have all the answers necessary to prevent it. At the current state of the art, physicians are able to slow the aging process and to significantly reverse many of the symptoms. Supplementing hormones as their levels decline is one of the most effective methods for reversing the symptoms of aging and improving your quality of life.

Hormone therapy and regulation is not simple since it affects our physiology in many ways. It should be undertaken only under the care of a physician knowledgeable in the nature of these hormones and their interactions, and who will monitor not only their levels but their effect on all aspects of your well-being.

Hormone therapy should accompany all of the other lifestyle improvements I've told you about in this book, especially in the areas of nutrition, exercise, and stress reduction. When you combine all of these lifestyle changes, the benefits will be life-altering. Comprehensive programs such as the ones offered by the Cenegenics Medical Institute are currently being quietly enjoyed by thousands of people around the world, very likely including a close friend or relative of yours!

twelve
live cell therapy:
the future of age management?

n the first chapter, I promised to cover the basics of age management and also to cover cutting-edge therapies that are considered to be the future in this field. Live cell therapy or *organotherapy* fits into this category. It shows amazing promise in its ability to rebuild and regenerate aging cells. What I tell you in this chapter comes from firsthand experience as a user of live cell technology.

I have experienced an array of benefits from this therapy. These benefits include a striking increase in the weight I am able to lift, a very rapid rebuilding of bone in my gums following dental surgery, and—if you'll excuse me for getting very personal, but in the interest of full disclosure of benefits—a powerful improvement in the strength and duration of my erections.

While live cell therapy may be further up the ladder of age intervention than you are interested in at this time, my role as your age-management guide is to keep you appraised of what is available. You (and your health care practitioner or physician) can decide what is right for you.

Live cell therapy is a method to revitalize the organs of the body—to bring new life where age and degenerative processes have robbed the cell of some of its size or some of its vital life-giving activities. Cell degeneration as we age is a very naturally occurring process according to some, and very unnatural according to the scientists who are looking into ways of preventing this process. As you know, I believe we should utilize as many medical advancements and miracles of science as are available to keep our cells healthy and young.

But to discuss this revitalization, which is really what organo-therapy is designed to do, you must understand the basic terms of cell aging. *Chronological* age doesn't stop with the passing of time; it just goes on as the clock ticks away, day in and day out. But *biological* age and vitality require a different definition. According to German physician and scientist Dr. Hoffiker, "An organism's biological age refers to its functional capacities corresponding to the respective stage of the individual's life span."

Now what is Dr. Hoffiker really saying here? He is trying to draw the distinction between a cell's "projected, expected" age and the actual health of that cell at any point during the cell's life.

Let's take the American average, and say you are going to live to 75 to 77 years of age. We will call this your life span. Now we will take a look at an organism inside your body. While the organism may be 19 or 20 years of age, that organism may, for one reason or another, already have used half or more of its functional life. If its life span was intended to be 77 years, that cell has prematurely aged—its biological age is already nearly 40 years old.

Another German scientist, Dr. Beier, defines vitality as "a measurement of an organism's ability to realize all its vital functions." Now if this cell is going to realize all of its vital functions, then it has to *perform* all of its vital functions. If it is not performing, then it has lost its vitality. And if it is already halfway through its biological life span, but only a third of the way through its projected chronological life span, then it is old before its time. When you see people who look old before their time, you can bet that millions of cells in their bodies are experiencing this process.

The poster child for this premise could be any one of a number of aging rock stars whose lifestyle of drugs, alcohol, and general abuse of their body is now coming home to roost. I don't mean to be insulting, but mental pictures can be powerful for demonstration purposes. Several of these musicians look decades older than their chronological age. Whatever they have done to the cells in their bodies, you can be sure that their intended life span is not being realized in any way, shape, or form.

Live cell therapy seeks to strengthen cells so they will go in the opposite direction from this example. Speaking of the promise of live cell therapy, Dr. Bier points out that "Revitalization is maintenance over an extended period, or the regaining of lost vitality in the latter years of life—after the climax—which significantly belongs to a younger biological age than the chronological age as objectified by several age parameters." But he adds, "The revitalizing effect of live cell therapy has been largely objectivated in animal experiments. In humans, this effect has been proven empirically on many patients. But, as of yet, results from coordinated clinical studies are lacking, due to the enormous difficulties in carrying out these studies."

As you know, I push the envelope when it comes to reversing aging. I don't want to get old waiting for ways to prevent me from getting old. You may be more conservative, and wish to wait for more clinical studies before you adopt live cell therapy into your age-management plan. But I want you to have the choice—the informed choice.

TAKE CONTROL OF THE CLOCK IN YOUR CELLS

You have organisms in your body that have a life span and a clock built into them somewhere. The problem is that the life span built into the cell and the life span that the cell is actually living out is frequently two different numbers.

For example, automobile manufacturers count on a happy medium. They believe that individuals who buy their cars are going to give them average maintenance. So the car is going to stay on the road approximately 10 years. However, one individual buys the car and really fools them. He changes the oil every time it is supposed to be changed, steam cleans the engine, makes sure that the shocks are always maintained so the car doesn't receive any unnecessary stress on the highway, and keeps new tires on it. He keeps the upholstery clean so grit and grime don't eat away at it, polishes the car, protects it with wax so wind and rain don't create rust or corrosion, and does complete regular maintenance. Ten years down the road, that car is almost as good as the day it came off the assembly line. It looks and performs almost like a brand-new car.

Then you may have another individual who buys the same model of car. But this individual drives the car into the ground. Instead of changing the oil every 3,000 miles, he changes it at 10,000 or 15,000 miles. He never changes the shocks until the car falls down on the frame. He waits for blowouts on the tires, never washes or polishes the car so the finish is rusted and corroded. Repairs and regular maintenance aren't part of his program. He never does anything about the upholstery and the carpets on the floor are wretched. In about four years, this car has had it. Nobody but nobody would buy this car.

So it has to go into a total "revitalization" stage, where someone has to take the car in and completely redo it. They have to bring in new metal to fill in where it is rusted and corroded. They have to pack it in, rub it out, blend it together, and polish it. Then they have to replace the upholstery, put in new shocks, a new driveshaft, and all the other parts to make that car function properly. They have to revitalize that car to bring it back and make it presentable.

Now let's apply the same possibilities to your body. Your cells and your organisms were designed to live out a certain life span. You have two choices. You can just go along and feed your body whatever it thinks it wants, or whatever it likes. You can abuse your body with cigarettes and alcohol and other environmental toxins. You can speed up that biological clock even ahead of the chronological clock to where that body of yours may not even last the expected life span of 75 or 77 years. Each organ inside will be really, really old for its age. However, it's still not too late to decide to take care of that body, even though it may have gone a little bit south on you or decayed a little bit. As the ultimate manager of your aging, you can choose to intervene at the cellular level.

INTERVENE WITH AGING AT THE CELLULAR LEVEL

AGE ERASER

One of the most potentially powerful ways to revitalize aging cells is through live cell therapy. In this innovative process, "like" cells are taken from certain animals (usually porcine or ovine) in the embryonic stages of development. The cells are extracted in the early stages—approximately the second month of pregnancy. They are not from more developed unborn animal fetuses where you might have the risk of viruses or other unwanted foreign substances.

In the porcine and ovine embryonic stage, there are striking similarities at the basic cellular level with many cells in human organs—similarities in the cellular signals transferred and messages that are carried by each cell. This premise will definitely be questioned and challenged—and that is fine. That's what science is all about. But I am choosing—having used this therapy myself and having experienced remarkable results—to believe that there is more fact than fiction here. And even though this therapy is in the early stages of development in the United States, it has been used for many, many years in Europe and other countries around the world by the very wealthy who could afford it.

In live cell therapy, the cells that are extracted from the embryonic stage of the developing porcine and ovine fetus have the development of all of their genetic growth and all of their message centers ahead of them. The cells are extracted in a very microbiotic way. They are processed in a GMP government approved lab.

The human body absorbs these cells, which then travel directly to their "organ counterpart" in the body. The cells have their own guidance system that directs them to the "like" organ from which the cells were harvested. Example: brain cells that are taken from the embryonic stage go directly to the brain. Cells from the adrenal gland go to the adrenal glands. The same is true for cells from the heart, liver, kidneys, spleen, testicles, ovaries, pancreas, and muscle tissue. No physiological action takes place until the tissue hooks up or docks up where it belongs in the human body. This is akin to DNA activity—nucleic acid behavior within the cell. The DNA has its own guidance system. It does not make mistakes inside your body.

Live cell therapy is the phenomenon of nature that we have never been able to duplicate. We always want to direct something one way or the other in the body. We want to put it where we think it belongs. But DNA has its own brain. When this lyophilized (freeze-dried) tissue comes into your body, no action takes place until it circulates through your system, goes up against the organ that it was designed to someday itself become, and latches on to the cell. Then it revitalizes the partnered cell with its yet-to-be-utilized life-span code—bringing life, stamina, and vitality back into the organism to which it has attached. A new support system for that cell has been created, because the live cell takes on the characteristics of the cell to which it has attached.

It is like sending a fresh running back into an NFL huddle. After you've utilized one running back to grind down the defense for three quarters, you send someone in who hasn't played all day. He has fresh, strong legs and all of his power is yet to be unleashed. All of a sudden, the defense is dealing with somebody who is brand spanking new and who is operating at optimum levels. He has not been beaten down; he is not tired.

Now think of that team getting ready for the next play. Over 90 percent of it is exactly the same as it was, but now, one player is different, and that creates a whole different team in terms of potential effectiveness and performance. This is exactly what happens in a human cell when the new live cell is introduced to it.

THINK BEYOND HORMONE REPLACEMENT

One of the important therapies you will read about in this book is hormone replacement therapy. And, as I have mentioned, in our company we prefer to *stimulate* your body to produce its own hormones at the levels it did somewhere in the early 20s. In both cases, you are increasing hormone levels to help direct your cells to function at optimum levels.

Live cell therapy goes a step further—it literally brings new building blocks into your body to rejuvenate your cells. This is why I call live cell therapy the next level of age management. It actually gives your body healthy cell-building materials—proteins and peptides that come into your body as a pure nitrogen type of protein in its finest form. They have already gone through all the right stages that you would hope to obtain from eating all the right foods in order to help you recycle and regenerate. The new cells dock up against your current cells and give them an infusion of youthful vitality.

If you think of your hormones as the architects and bricklayers directing and executing the construction of your cells and organs, the live cells are like fresh new mortar being brought in by a convoy of shiny, new trucks. The trucks are bringing in actual cell tissue—the material that can grow and can expand and interweave with your cells to help them come back to a more youthful size and capacity. Hormone therapy will provide stimulation, but your cells need the new materials and the building blocks to actually become younger.

These live cells come into your body and introduce very "like" material into your own cells. Your brain is going to tell each cell what to do after it becomes part of your tissue. Your bloodstream and your DNA will take over. To answer a question I hear frequently, "No, you are not operating under the DNA of an animal." You are only receiving the benefits of the transference process—similar to energy and nutrition you receive when you eat a thick, juicy steak. All that this lyophilized live cell material understands is that it is to latch on and to grow, and it becomes part of your original cell.

If you adopt a child, it comes from a different set of parents. But if you adopted the child as an infant, even though it may have different genetics, over the next 15 to 20 years, that child, under your guidance and with its relationship with all its new little brothers and sisters, will be a part of your family as much as anybody else. The adopted child will function, if treated like the rest of the children, like the rest of the family.

I did a television show not long ago at the famous Steadman-Hawkins Sports Medicine Clinic, where athletes such as John Elway, Greg Norman, Monica Seles, and Picabo Street have gone for surgery and rehabilitation. Dr. Steadman showed me the marvelous things that they could do by opening bone up and leaving just enough of a gap so the bone and marrow can regenerate and regrow itself to fill in the gap. They have now learned that they can regenerate tissue, something they didn't believe they could do before. Live cell therapy is on the cutting edge of this new world of cell regeneration.

I recently had some bone surgery on the roof of my mouth. The doctors were amazed how rapidly the bone in my jaw grew back. At the time, I was using live cells of additional bone marrow and cartilage. My new bone grew back three times faster than they were used to seeing. The process that they were using—mineralized human bone tissue—was normally taking at least 90 days for bone to form, heal, and grow to quarter of an inch thickness. In less than 40 days, my bone had completely filled in. This is what you can do when you have the proper building blocks. And live cell therapy brings that to your body. It creates an incredible revitalization if used as part of your entire age-management program.

TREAT EVERY PART OF YOUR BODY TO LIVE CELLS

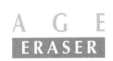

Live cell therapy comes in the form of organic dietary supplements in 31 different extracts including: adrenal, artery, bone marrow, brain, cartilage, eye, gall bladder, intestine, kidney, heart, hypothalamus, ligament, liver, lung, mesenchyme, muscle, ovaries, pancreas, pituitary, prostate, spinal, placenta, spleen, stomach, testicle, gonad, thymus, thyroid, veins, and vessels.

You literally choose the part of your body that your are trying to enhance. That is exactly what I have done, and I'm going to take you through the components of this program that I have utilized and the results that I have achieved.

Most people who know me know that I love to train with weights. And as we weight lifters get older, we strive to maintain muscle mass and strength. My strength has always been at the upper echelon because I've always pushed the limits during my workouts.

I will give you a couple examples of what happened to my weight training, and then I will tell you which live cells I took. I was doing my leg presses on a leg press machine. I normally do these in 5 sets. I normally do 12 to 15 reps, then 10 to 12 reps, then 8 to 10 reps, then 6 to 8 reps and I usually finish my last set with 4 to 6 reps. In my last set, I had worked up to 1050 pounds. After 6 weeks on live cell therapy, my leg presses had increased from 1050 pounds to 1600 pounds—and I was doing a set of 4 to 5 repetitions. My squats increased 35 percent. My dumbbell presses on the flat bench went from 110 pounds with each hand to 150 pounds, an incredible elevation of about 40 percent. My recovery system and aerobic capacity became phenomenal. My duration increased dramatically on the treadmill and on the cross-trainer, and I wasn't even breathing hard.

What Was I Taking?

I did several things that I believe in. One of my great energy sources was adrenal—I've always believed in the power of that gland's energy rush. And since I was performing great load-bearing exercises, I added bone marrow to my program. Obviously, I wanted to improve my mental acuity, so I took the brain cells as part of my package. I would alternate weeks with the bone marrow and the cartilage. I took the hypothalamus, because I wanted the hypothalamic activity within my body to keep my thyroid (my heat control thermostat) and everything within my system working properly. I took the ligament because I wanted to strengthen my ligaments and tendons. I took it on alternate weeks with the mesenchyme, because the mesenchyme works in a similar fashion in the joints and provides tremendous ligament and tendon strength.

I never took the muscle because I consume enough protein, and didn't feel my muscles needed any more help at that point. I took the thymus to build up my immune function and primary regulation of the immune responses. And I took the pituitary throughout the entire program to make sure the activity in my pituitary gland continued to help me keep my IGF-1 levels up and active.

I took the placenta, along with the testicle and the gonad, for my libido. Personal details here are not necessary, but suffice to say, the therapy worked. The testicle cells are very important because they increase and improve male hormone functions, balancing them out and helping to increase sexual functions. I also alternated weeks between the arteries and the veins live cells. I wanted the increased circulation, and I think this had a lot to do with the improved blood flow between the elevated libido in my brain and the required performance level of my sexual organs.

These are the cells that I took, and I experienced some very positive results. Any of the extracts in live cell therapy can be taken with any of the others, and each will relate to the organ from which it is derived. But make no mistake, this is relatively new science. It may or may not be for everybody. However, I do believe it is worth a serious look. People ask if their health care professionals will have knowledge about this therapy, and at this point, the answer is probably that only doctors who are versed in antiaging or age-management medicine will be able to direct you. In the future, my company, in conjunction with Jean Berry and Life Cell Technologies, will host educational training seminars. We will also include much of this information in our Forever Young newsletter, both print and online.

In writing about this innovative therapy, I have obviously spoken from the male perspective. I'm a man. I've used this therapy. I have been able to tell you from intimate knowledge what specific type of cells I used, why I used them, and what I experienced or what had changed after the therapy. I have given you the firsthand case history of a male experience.

Live cell therapy can be just as valuable to women. I do not have the authority to speak from firsthand use as a woman, of course, but I *have* spoken to many women who have used the therapy successfully. Women have reported increased strength, greater skin elasticity, a lessening of lines and wrinkles, and greater muscle density that helped eliminate pockets of fat throughout their body.

Osteoporosis is certainly a nemesis of the aging female (and the aging male, we are now discovering). Mesenchyme cell therapy is particularly effective against osteoporosis and some arthritis in the hands, fingers, knees, and back. Placenta, pituitary, and thymic have also proven very effective at stimulating and improving women's immune system.

Live cell therapy works essentially the same for women as men, with difference in only the gender-specific live cells. And again, even though these cells are taken from animals, they interact safely and efficiently with humans.

Are There Any Contraindications?

It is always best to consult with your health care practitioner or physician. However, as a dietary supplement, live cell therapy is the same as consuming other food supplements in an extremely concentrated form. These are proteins at the highest level. People want to know how this fits into taking vitamins, minerals, or protein supplements. Live cell supplements are designed to be easily assimilated, absorbed, and used by the body so the body will benefit in many ways, maintaining its function and structure when rebuilding organs. It works very well with your vitamins, minerals, and antioxidants. It certainly does not work against them, and it should enhance the output of each and every one.

Should These Be Taken If You Have a Disease?

As with any therapy, use great caution and ask your doctor's advice if you suffer from any disease whatsoever. Live cell supplements are not currently sold as pathology for any disease.

Are There Any Negative Side Effects?

I know of none, and have certainly experienced none myself. The products I have been associated with are taken orally in a sublingual manner. All supplements should improve the quality of your life, as they are designed to maintain and strengthen your body structure and your body function. However, since this is not a program that is under the guidelines or the regulations of the FDA (since it is classified as a food supplement, not a drug), I would always recommend that you research this for yourself and ask your medical practitioner to review it with you.

I choose to take control of my body. I intend to stop the clock. I intend to turn the clock back. These are my decisions; they are not going to be made for me by the FDA or anyone else. I am not against the FDA.

It is there for a purpose—to protect you from harmful drugs. I do not consider these to be drugs, let alone harmful. But I would strongly suggest that if you do make your own decisions regarding new therapies, then you must take the time to become as informed and educated as possible.

Read everything that you can read. Be cautious. Don't go overboard taking an abundance of anything. And consult with your physician. Remember, I get my blood tested every 8 to 12 weeks. If something even begins to go wrong in my body, I am in a position and time frame to correct it.

If you are a woman who could become pregnant, I strongly suggest that you consult and review this therapy with your physician before beginning. It may be that your physician will tell you to continue the therapy if it was begun before pregnancy, but not to start it after you have conceived; or not to continue it beyond a specific month of pregnancy. This is an issue that should be discussed thoroughly between you and your health care practitioner.

Live cell therapy is not something I am telling you to go out and do. It is something I am telling you is worth looking into. And, again, if you make the decision to explore and perhaps try this therapy, make sure you educate yourself as much as you possibly can on the subject and that you are comfortable with your decision. This is the only way to make certain that you are doing the right thing—for you.

Where Can I Get Live Cell Therapy Products?

Seek only the finest live cells on the market. Make sure they were extracted in the embryonic stage using the lyophilized process. I trust only one source at this time. I get my products from a company in Coconut Grove, Florida, called Life Cell Technologies International. The company is owned by a women in her 70s named Jean Berry, who is absolutely an incredible picture of health and vitality. Anyone who sees her youthful appearance and energy wants to know what she does to stay so young. It is quite obvious to me that Jean uses her own products and practices what she preaches. She has done this for many years and is an extraordinary woman with an enormous amount of vitality. She is also a perfectionist who has traveled the globe meeting personally with the physicians and looking at the labs and facilities where all the development of the Life Cell Technologies products takes place. She has even visited the farms where the animals are raised. That's why Life Cell

Technologies is the only source I would use to procure live cell products that I intend to put into my body. See the reference section at the end of the book for contact information.

OPEN YOUR MIND AND BODY TO NEW WAYS TO REVERSE AGING

Live cell therapy is one of the things that you can do to restructure and rebuild your cells. Whether you are a doctor, lawyer, runner, weight lifter, stay-at-home mom, or businessperson—it doesn't matter what you do or who you are—you are living life and damaging cells. Those cells need to be regenerated and revitalized, and I believe live cell therapy is an excellent way to do it.

Live cell therapy is something that I believe in. But I am not saying that it is the be-all and end-all. Hormone replacement therapy, vitamins, minerals, herbs, and antioxidants aren't the exclusive answers either. All of these, including exercise, proper rest, reading of spiritually guiding material, and more go into age management—the process of slowing it down. It is being done on a daily basis by many and you can do it too. You can begin with this book, and by doing your homework.

You can choose not to accept the things that I have to say here—and that is perfectly all right. My purpose for writing this book is not to have you buy into every single word that I write or procedure that I utilize in my life. My objective is to get you to think about it. I want you to think about your mortality and your ability to manage when and how you arrive at that distant point.

Your genetic process is influenced continually by a series of biological processes and subcellular changes that you go through during your life. You experience extracellular changes, tissue alterations, and impaired abilities in organs that affect the actual specific functions that are intended to be carried out in your body. As time goes by, your health and longevity, in turn, are negatively affected by the diminished adaptability to the elements that attack your body—by the free radical systems that reduce and shut it down. All of this works together to increase the possibility of sickness, premature aging, and death.

Of course this is inevitable, but the question is, *when* is it inevitable? Through organotherapy, along with other techniques discussed in this book, we are able to revitalize our cells. We are able to restimulate the molecules and—right at the molecular level—we are able to develop organ tissue, to strengthen tissue, and to increase the functional capacity of our system. The population of cells now is performing at more optimal levels. Our outward vitality is a direct mirror of the performance level of the hundreds of millions of tiny molecular structures in our body.

That's what is important. The physiological parameters that go on inside your body are what you reflect outside your body. You have to accept some of these things as being true, whether or not you accept every methodology that might correct the process. When you understand what is taking place inside your body, you may choose to do something about it. If this book stimulates you to reach out for that greater vitality, you can push that mortality rate way beyond the sunset of what others expect it to be. You will be able to be 60, 70, and 80 years of age and do all of the things you did in your 20s.

Believe me, I tell you this as a matter of record—a fact of my life and the lives of hundreds of people who choose to live this way. These people are in their late 50s and 60s—and some are in their 70s and 80s. They are the Jack LaLannes of the world who do the things that others have given up. Why have they given up? Because they believe that they *can't* do things. Because they've allowed themselves to buy into that *can't* theory. A long time ago they decided to let their bodies go, and now, even with all that's available in science and medicine, they cannot allow themselves to believe it can be turned around.

You *can* turn it around, but you have to get rid of the word *can't* and replace it with the words *can* and *will*. How? By opening up your mind, your heart, your spirit, and your body and making the decision to take control of the way you age. Take control of your life span. Existing is *not* living. I want you to *live!*

thirteen
the ultimate age eraser:
you and your relationships

A wise person once said that the ultimate thrill is in the journey, not the destination. Friends have recently said to me, "Wow, you must be really excited about finally becoming an author!" As I reflected on some of the great authors I've read over the years, I certainly could not put myself in their category—neither my ego nor my education would permit me to do so. Rather than an author, I see myself as a scientist of sorts. A scientist is, in my opinion, someone who is willing to experiment, to reach for and then possibly try the unknown.

This doesn't mean that I want you to use your body to test all sorts of strange and unknown chemicals. What I am saying is that throughout my lifetime, having been privy to great information and having worked with wonderful physicians and scientists, I have been willing to experiment—to utilize my body to see what positive changes could be made. I have tried the therapies that I believed could possibly affect my energy levels, my sleep patterns, my personality, or my moods. Would a specific experiment create mood swings, and would I always have a positive attitude? In the same manner I have used my body to experiment with different exercises and their specific effects on muscle tone, muscle strength, flexibility, and stamina. This is the way I have chosen to use *my* body.

So I have always seen myself as an amateur scientist in this field more than anything else. But in order to write this book and share the knowledge I gained through my personal experiences, I also had to see myself as a reporter of events past and present. This has only been reaffirmed as writing of this book progressed.

During the past 50-some-odd years, there have been many people who contributed to my life's journey to this point. There are many physicians, many athletes, many celebrities, and so many people from various walks of life who have always been kind and generous enough to share their time and their thoughts with me. I feel privileged to have received information from others, but also honored that they allowed me to express my thoughts and ideas to them. To me, this is the basis upon which to build an honest and solid relationship.

I have always enjoyed establishing new relationships. Our life's relationships are such an invaluable part of us that they may, in fact, be the ultimate age erasers. And there are so many varieties of relationships. Just as your body has trillions of cells in it with many different jobs and duties to carry out, with each and every cell providing something very specialized to your existence, so the various relationships in your lifetime contribute to who you become. No one person, no one event, no one thing, epitomizes everything that you *are*, everything that you *will* be, or everything that you *can* be. Each and every relationship along your journey through life has contributed—some in small ways, some in major ways—to who you are, to what you are, to how you think, to your desires, to your goals, and to your accomplishments.

The relationships I've had throughout my life have contributed in a huge way to the content of this book. I have been a very fortunate man. I have been able to share my life with a wonderful family, accounting somewhere along the way for the upbringing of seven children. I had a great woman who helped me do this. I had great friends. I had valuable associates. I have had the opportunity to walk many paths and form many great relationships.

I have also had the good fortune to be personally acquainted with some of the great athletes of our time, to work with them in their exercise and weight-training programs, and to share their psychological approach to their game. I've known major television personalities and many major motion picture actors and actresses along the way. I was given the opportunity to interview them, spend social time with them, spend professional time with them, and to hear their viewpoints. This included not just their "on the record" views for public consumption, but their private goals and motivations as well. We've also talked about the price they paid to become what their public persona is perceived to be. From these associations I learned what many famous people were like behind the scenes, and what relationships in their lives played a part in determining who they were, and what they would become.

The total accumulation of these friendships and relationships were in my mind as I worked my way through the pages of this book. Before there were pages in this book there were pages in my mind. These pages reflect my life experiences—experiences I've lived through and sifted through in order to share them here with you.

This book is subtitled *100 Age-Erasing Techniques,* and while I was writing the book, what excited me most was that each and every item I wrote about was something that I'd had the privilege to experience myself. This is why I call myself a scientist. Both my mind and my body have been a laboratory that I've used to collect and either validate or invalidate data gathered through my personal journey. Acting as a scientist, using my own mind and body, seeing the results, and then wanting to share what I've learned, has brought me to the present time where I am now ready to share all that I've learned—to put it all into print to be read by everyone I want to help.

In this book I have shared techniques or specific therapies that I have tried and applied, and in turn have watched others apply to their lives. I've seen people make great changes in their lives over the years by using some of the principles you've read about. But none of these are as potentially powerful as the relationships you will experience over a lifetime.

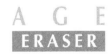

LOOK WITHIN YOURSELF

Up to this point we've talked about only the physical aspects of remaining Forever Young, but to build solid relationships we must now focus on the mental and spiritual aspects of remaining Forever Young. The mental aspect is perceived as being learned information and our conditioned response to that learned information. The spiritual aspect begins with your relationship with yourself.

Although I'm writing this book after 59-plus years of real and practical experience out in the world, having done everything I could to remain active and also to help as many people as I could to enjoy the same benefits, I also realize that behind everything I've done there was a strong spiritual driving force. This force was instilled in me from the day I was born by a very religious mother, who gave me a rather strict Roman Catholic upbringing. Now, I know that not everyone reading this book has the same religious background—be it Roman Catholic, or Jewish, or Buddhist, or Muslim, or any of the multitudes of spiritual backgrounds shared by people all over the world today. In fact, it isn't really important whether or not you practice *any* organized religion.

As a result of sending good wishes to a friend of mine during a recent Christian holiday, I received a return e-mail from him reminding me that he was an atheist. I knew that, but I was extending to him my good wishes anyway. While reminding me of his atheism, he also expressed a very positive thought, saying that he had noticed the positive aspects brought to many of his friend's lives by their various faiths. He noticed the good feelings they seemed to experience in the practice of their faiths. Although he was not willing to accept any particular religion, he certainly was appreciative of the positive effects enjoyed by many practitioners. And his comments are basically what I am trying to say to you here in this chapter.

In *my* life, my *personal* life, God provided for me that major chamber of my mind where I could go when there was nowhere else to turn. But religion does not necessarily have to be your motivator. It may be a particular event in your life—or a particular person or a specific goal. It may be something that you take out of a conscious state and put into a subconscious state so it is there to constantly remind you, drive you, or bring you back to center. It enables you—it motivates you so that you are finally able to accomplish something that has eluded you in the past.

All great accomplishments have not come from great people. Many extraordinary things have been done by very ordinary people. I hope that this book, coming from a very ordinary man, will perhaps result in some extraordinary events in other ordinary lives. I want to remind all of us that we live in a world where we suffer so many maladies that cause death, disability, and simple daily fatigue and illness—all the things, large and small, that prevent us from experiencing the joy and positive nature of life on this earth. We talk about serious illnesses like cancer, coronary disease, and cardiovascular disease, but one thing that has really caught my attention is the incredible rise of stress factors in our lives.

Everything we do, beginning even as a child competing in sports for fun, recreation, and exercise, brings with it the stress of feeling that we must succeed. At a young age we already feel the pressure to be better than our peers, to satisfy our mom and dad or our coach. We are already trying to live up to others' expectations, and the minute we begin to do this we begin to experience stress.

Then comes the pressure to succeed academically on increasingly difficult levels, so that we will be seen as employable. If we are lucky, we get that job and begin to experience life in the real world. Then we find out what *real* pressure is all about as we struggle to succeed in our chosen profession. If we own our business, there is even more pressure and stress. Whether as employee or employer, we experience the need to succeed and the subsequent pressures of delivering what is expected of us, getting projects in on time, and meeting deadlines.

And then there is what may be the most important source of stress in our life today: being a good father or mother to our children. Our children face so many more potential complications in their lives than we did. They are forced to deal with exposure to many forms of substance abuse, and they are exposed via television and other media to so much more of life's difficult realities. Our children are not necessarily given the viewpoint that life as an adult is a wonderful thing to look forward to, and, in fact, sometimes they are shown that life may not be worth living. This is such a tragedy because we as human beings are the greatest miracle of all. Living life fully is truly an amazing experience.

If you live every day of that journey, you will not let one day go by that you do not try to find a piece of happiness or to accomplish something that makes *you* happy. Yes, you! You're not here on earth to please everyone else, you are here to please one person—you. Because once you please *you*, you'll have the capability to begin to please others. I'll talk more about pleasing yourself later in this chapter with a quote from a poem that pretty well expresses what you have to do for yourself. Because stress is the great killer, *and most stress comes from within.*

And that's where the tragedy begins, because it is the pressure we place on ourselves, the expectations that we have of ourselves that cause the most stress and damage from stress. And most of that stress wouldn't be there if we didn't allow others to influence us. You say to yourself, "Someone thinks I should do this, someone thinks I should do that," and then you begin to tell yourself, "Oh my gosh, I need to do this, I need to do that, but I don't have the time, I don't have the resources, I don't have the talent to do that—why do they think I can do it?" Pretty soon your whole world is stressed out. You have nowhere to go and no one to talk to. You're a bundle of nerves. Your blood pressure rises. This is where people develop strokes; this is where diabetes sometimes comes in. You'd be amazed at what stress can do, and yes, stress can literally create impotency in your life, and I'm sure you don't want that!

So when I talk to you about looking inside yourself, when I talk to you about where I go—that refreshing place where I go to calm my nerves, to eliminate stress—I'm not saying that you need to go to the same place, that you need to find solace and inspiration in your religion. You just have to accept and understand that you need to go *somewhere* mentally, to be with something that is inside of you. You need to find out where or what allows you to get your mind and your focus off of what is causing you stress, and put yourself in the presence of that calming influence. Stress kills. Stress hinders what you can do with your life. Eliminate it.

I often go to songs. Music often possesses a great calming effect that allows you to lose yourself for a while, away from your worries or your concerns. If you choose upbeat music you just might find yourself singing along! Just be cautious about your music choices—turning on a "somebody done me wrong" country tune might not be the best choice. But it's ultimately your choice as to what music does the most for you. Make a good choice and listen to something that lifts your spirit. Find something personal that motivates you out of any ill will, out of any bad feelings, out of mental fatigue, out of physical fatigue, out of depression, out of all that yucky stuff in life.

When I hear songs, I wonder if the writers were inspired by another human being they might be sharing their love with, or if they are perhaps inspired by, or seeking to attach themselves to, some higher spiritual element outside of themselves that they might not fully understand.

I know that in our daily lives we sometimes feel let down by others because they are not meeting our expectations—our *false* expectations—that they should live up to *our* standards. But remember this about relationships: it is not what you receive *from* them, but what you give *to* them. Because you're never ever going to be able to give more than you receive. If you'll just keep on giving, you'll be amazed at what you receive.

If you have not already, I promise you that one day soon you will reach a point in your life where you will need to talk to someone who can answer your questions, solve your problems, and another human being won't be able to help. They just won't understand. They will have their own set of problems. Then you've got to go not outside, but inside of yourself. You've got to go inside your spiritual world to get the answers. You need to have someone or something to answer your questions. You need somewhere to go—some chamber of your mind where you find solace, find something to believe in, find some psychological relief that will allow you to go on.

For me, the person to go to was God. Whether you go to Allah, Mohammed, a rabbi, or a priest—whatever your spiritual leader may be called—the only thing I call upon you to have is some kind of spiritual relationship with something or someone beyond yourself, for those moments when you just don't have all the answers.

We've all been there. We've all come to that point where we feel no one understands us, that we have a very unique problem, that there's no one we can talk to because no one can understand *our* problem. Well, if you have nowhere to go you will never have an answer. If you have no one to give that up to, you are never, ever going to be able to fully resolve your problems.

We are going to talk about the relationships you have with loved ones in your life. We are going to talk about the relationship you may have with your spouse, with your children, with your partner, with your employer, with your friends, with the world around you, but most importantly the relationship you have with yourself. What expectations do you have of yourself? How much control do you feel you have over your relationships? How much control do you want to have? How much do you want to give up to someone else? These are the questions that everyone ponders.

I can hear you saying to me, "Bill, I don't want any more questions, I want some answers!" Well, I told you that I pray *to* God, I didn't say that I *was* God. You'll have to learn how to get inside yourself—how to realize that there is a spirit living within you that guides everything that you do. I'm not sure what you'll call it. Some people say they're guided by their conscience. But what is that conscience? It's what tells you the difference between what is right and what is wrong. Well then, what *is* right and what *is* wrong?

If you live in a remote jungle in Africa, what is considered right or wrong might be a little different than what is considered right or wrong in Manhattan. Your methods of survival might be a little bit different. Your way of communicating might be different. Your ways of purchasing things, including information, might be different, whether it is by barter or trading or just having the cold, hard cash. So where do you go to get the answers? And is there just one set of answers? Yes, there is. But that set of answers is unique to you. There *is* one answer because the one answer is always inside of *you*, the individual. And you won't come up with the same answer I come up with, or the same answer your spouse comes up with, and so on.

I deal with relationships in light of who I perceive myself to be. You deal with them in light of your own self-perception. This is the first point in trying to understand the great age eraser that human relationships are. To understand you and your relationships, you must understand your relationship with yourself. You must understand your self-image—how you see yourself, what you believe about yourself, and what you believe you were meant to be.

Do you see yourself as a good person, a bad person, a smart person, someone who enjoys life, or someone who sees the worst in everyone? Are you judgmental, and yet want no one to judge you? Are you a person who simply lives day to day with no opinion about anything or anyone, figuring that all life will take care of itself? I don't know whether any of these are the way you see yourself. But I can tell you that the one thing in life that will guarantee your failure is the inability to have a satisfying relationship with yourself.

Just for a moment, imagine the best person you can create, the finest person you can design, with the best of all characteristics. I'm not speaking of physical appearance. I'm speaking of character makeup—someone whose actions, words, and deeds are the best you can imagine. Mentally create that person, and reflect on it just for a moment. Now put your name on that person. Make that person *you*. Why not? Didn't you just design that person to perfection? Isn't that *who* and *what* you thought would comprise the best someone could be?

I'm not asking you to accept my God. I'm not asking you to select any particular faith or buy into any belief of mine or of anyone else. I am asking you to take a strong look at yourself and maximize the benefits of the power that you have over your own universe.

How many times have you heard that perception becomes reality? It only becomes a reality because you let it be so. As we perceive circumstances, so our mind reacts to what we believe to be true. Whether it is actually true or not isn't important.

Before beginning a painting or a building, an artist has a *vivid* picture already in his mind and an architect *sees* a structure in his mind. They both decide ahead of time what *they* want the painting and the building to look like. They both have *clear pictures* of what *they* want to see before putting paint or pencil to paper.

If you are going to be the architect of your life, if you want to establish positive, harmonious relationships with others, you must begin by establishing one with yourself. You must find peace with who and what you are. You must feel confident about what you can accomplish. You must feel confident about your achievements and grateful for the talents that you have. You must begin to maximize your talents. To do this you must understand the first rule of all, that you must actually love yourself. Disregard what anyone may say about this being self-serving. It is exactly that. It *is* self-serving. You must serve yourself a dose of love every single day. You must allow yourself to love yourself because you are not going to take care of anything or anybody that you do not first love. You cannot give love to others that you do not have within yourself. So make a point to wake up every morning and look in the mirror and say "I love you" to the person looking back. You think it sounds silly, try it for five or six days. Tell yourself "I love you and today we're going out and accomplish something." You will be amazed at what happens to you in the next five or six days. You will be amazed about how much better you feel about yourself and how your mental and physical health will improve. So make your first rule of the day to tell yourself that you are loved—by you!

The reason I've talked so much about good health in this book is because the better you feel, the better you'll look, and the better you'll function and conduct yourself. It's very simple: if you are going to operate at the top of your game you're going to need to be the best that you can possibly be. And this will all become reality if you realize that your first love is for yourself. That will give you plenty of love to give to anyone else.

When NASCAR drivers are preparing for the Daytona 500 or any of the other grueling races on the circuit, the mechanics are out there working their tails off, building a tremendous frame for the car, making sure the mechanicals, the electricals, and the safety devices are all in top condition. They are doing everything that is humanly possible to make the car they are working on as safe, as powerful, and as effective as it possibly can be. But they must have one more vital ingredient: a driver in peak condition, one who can withstand 500 miles of grueling, heat-intense racing.

There aren't too many moments to relax when you're driving around a track at 200 mph with only a sheet of metal separating you from 40 other cars. A driver must be in peak condition to give his best and do justice to the machine and, I might add, to himself. After all, top condition in a situation like this just might save your life.

Well, to do justice to your life and to every event that you're going to be involved in, you too must be in peak physical condition, peak mental condition, and have the needed spiritual support for your system. I call it spiritual. I don't care what you call it. It is simply something inside you, a belief system to take you where you need to go when the world doesn't have the answers and you're ready to give up.

Call it faith or call it spirituality. Call it metaphysical. I don't care. I'm not trying to impress upon you my particular faith or belief system. Successful and harmonious relationships are not accidents. They are thought out and planned. They are worked for and achieved. And everything in life is achieved a lot easier when your relationship with yourself is a good one. If *you* like *you*, it makes it a lot easier to like someone else.

If you believe in you, you'll believe that if a relationship is worth having, it is worth giving it everything you've got. And you'll believe that every time you have a relationship with someone it is improved because *you* are a part of it. Because you've got a lot to give! If you believe that you've got a lot to give and if you apply this to every one of your relationships, what a wonderful life you'll have!

How many times have you heard the story of a man and a woman in a relationship whose love is burning strong long after their golden wedding anniversary? They do everything together. They shop together. They take walks together. They like the same television shows, movies, and plays. They count on each other in every aspect of their lives. Then, sadly, one of them takes ill and passes on. Soon, the remaining partner who was in very vibrant health seems to decline. In a very short period of time their health slips away, and pretty soon they have gone to join their mate.

When I hear these stories I often wonder if it's by design. How powerful is the mind? If you have been with someone for 50, 60, or 70 years and for some reason they are no longer in your life, can you *will* your way back to them? Can you absolutely just let yourself go and shut down your body clock? How powerful is love in a relationship?

I believe that a spiritual relationship is a key element in your quest to remain forever young. In a recent Duke University Medical Center study published in the *Journal of Gerontology*, researchers discovered that relatively healthy seniors, who said they rarely or never prayed, ran about a 50 percent greater risk of dying during the six-year study compared with seniors who prayed at least once a week.

I know the infusion of vitality that my relationship with my God gives me, but beyond this emotional lift, there are specific scientific benefits that come from an active spiritual life, whatever you may choose to call it. According to the researchers at Duke, prayer and meditation are known to reduce stress, which causes a stronger immune response. At an age when heart disease, cancer, arthritis, and an assortment of other debilitating diseases are so prevalent, the strength of one's immune response is a key indicator of longevity.

A good friend of mine recently told me about his father and his father-in-law. His 70-year-old father was constantly referring to himself as an old man. And everything about him was, in fact, tired and old. He moved slowly and weakly. He was often ill. He was always depressed and out of sorts, cranky, and dispirited. On the other hand, my friend's 74-year-old father-in-law was happy and active. He was industrious and involved with life. He dressed sharply, told jokes, painted houses, planted a garden, and was a pleasure to be around. He never talked about his age or, more important, *acted his age.*

What a difference an attitude about age can make! Somewhere the tired old man was made to believe that folks his age were supposed to just meekly run out the clock. Unfortunately, this is a belief held by millions of people. You see it everywhere in people who seem resigned to the *expected* pattern of declining health and vigor as they age. But my friend's father-in-law believed something else about aging. He was aging on *his* terms, and enjoying every single day.

So what's the connection here? Love, prayer, spirituality, individual belief, and relief systems—each has a profound influence on successful aging. Without mastery of these aspects of your life, the power of the first 12 chapters of this book will be severely diminished.

CONTROL YOUR ENVIRONMENT

First of all, let's talk about your relationship with the world around you and how you fit into it. What does your environment have to do with remaining Forever Young? It has little or nothing to do with it—or it has everything to do with it. It all depends on how you see yourself relating to your environment. Are you a victim of it, or are you in control? If you don't like your situation, do you get depressed and resign yourself to unhappiness? Or do you see everything as an opportunity to better your world and yourself? This is more than a philosophy. This is more than a theory in a self-help book or a prayer book.

Many spiritual leaders will tell you to put your problems in God's hands and it will be all right. I'm going to tell you that whoever or whatever your god is, or whether or not you even recognize a god, *those hands are your hands.* If you truly have a spiritual source, a higher power, if you understand spiritual awareness, you will realize that spirit walks, talks, and breathes within you. *You* are the master of your destiny. *You* are the person who decides exactly what your environment will be.

You've heard the expression "think globally, act locally." I'm going to employ this phrase to bring my philosophical beliefs about controlling your environment to a completely manageable level. The environment I'm referring to is all within the lining of the largest organ of your body—your skin. It is controlled and contained by your bones. It moves with the muscle you control. Your environment comes from within, and the one thing that you control is what goes on within your body—from the moment you will it to be well, to the moment that you support that will to be well by providing it with everything it *needs*.

Note—I did not say all the things that it *wants*. Don't confuse these terms! When you introduce something into your body, or engage in a certain behavior, is it really right for your universe? Have you decided this is what your body needs, or have you been swayed by a marketing and media culture that is motivated by factors other than your good health and longevity? What is it that controls you? If you are not happy with your health, your fitness level, or your appearance, why is that? Is it something outside of your control that has allowed this to happen? Then you haven't accepted my message yet.

What's the message? Although poets have expressed the message using flowery expressions about being the "master of their fate" and the "captain of their soul," it's really the simple idea that *you* must take control and responsibility for your actions and your life, that what *you* believe is what you will become, that what *you* focus on is what you will accomplish, that *you* must accept accountability for your thought processes, and that by doing so, *you* will control your life.

In my life I was blessed to be the guardian and the safekeeper of seven children. Somewhere along the paths of their lives, they have all heard me say, "The change, the decision making, doesn't take 30 days, it doesn't take a week, it doesn't even take 24 hours. If you don't like what you see, if you don't like what you are, you must make the decision to change." As the ad says, just do it!

You and only you can make that decision. And from that moment on, you will begin living your life the way you want to live it. It really is that simple. Make the decision to change your environment. If you physically found yourself someplace you didn't want to be, you'd leave, wouldn't you? You make the little changes for your momentary comfort, right? So make the big changes that affect your whole life.

And don't be afraid to try different roads. It's been said that if you risk nothing, you stand to lose everything. If you don't like one change you've made, try another. It's as easy as walking into a dark room where all you need to do is throw the switch and there will be light. You have to recognize not just who you've been, but who you want to be, and take the first step to becoming just that!

And what is it you want to become? I believe you must become a complete and whole universe all on your own. You must believe you are as complete and as good as you can be. Once you've done this, then and only then do you really have something worthwhile to share with someone else. It all begins with you. You are a self-contained universe who is now ready to share a relationship with another self-contained universe.

A G E
ERASER

TO THINE OWN SELF BE TRUE

Long before I walked on this earth, there lived a philosophical gentleman, a playwright, who could make you laugh or cry, whose name was William Shakespeare. Of the many famous lines that Mr. Shakespeare wrote to amuse us, to thrill us, and sometimes to confuse us, the one that is perhaps most often quoted is "To thine own self be true."

But what if we changed it just slightly and said, "To thy *known* self be true"? Think about it. Who do you know yourself to be? Who do you want to be? Deep inside you know, you just need to get comfortable with it. You are a miracle and you have much to offer all on your own. When you accept that, you can share with everyone you come in contact with the real and true you—the truly best you have to offer.

From time to time, an artist steps back from his canvas to reflect on the painting as a whole. If you want to really take control of your behavior, you too need to step back and attempt to understand what lies behind it. What are the motivations behind your behaviors and what are the belief systems that are framing your perceptions? Is someone else deciding what your perceptions are? Do you have a preconceived notion of how a person is supposed to act, look, and feel at 30, 40, 50, or 60? Are you tracing the steps of old stereotypes or blazing the way for new ones?

Do you think of a 50-plus person as someone who is pulling out his or her AARP card to get on a bus to go collect a Social Security check? Or do you think of 50-plus as Arnold Schwarzenegger (age 53) leaping from building to building in a big-screen action film, or Tina Turner (age 61) gyrating across the stage? A friend of mine, action hero and movie star Steven Seagal, who will soon be 50, still does all of his own fight scenes and stunts. He is capable of this because he not only practices the physical principles in this book, he believes in the power of the internal spirit we're speaking of here. As much as anyone I know, Steven has a total belief in who he really is.

Once you understand your beliefs, you will be able to master them. Or as Shakespeare might say, you can be true to them. What is the reality that you envision for yourself? Do you have the will and mental discipline to create it? Do you really believe that your relationship with the universe and the environment around you is within your control? Do you believe your relationship with yourself reflects the fact that you are living your life the way you want it to be lived?

If there is something that is stressing you out, if there is something that you dislike about yourself or something inside that you are not comfortable with, then you are in darkness. Cut it out and get rid of it! After all, your body is your house! If, in your home, you had an old piece of furniture or an appliance that no longer worked, wouldn't you get rid of it and replace it with a new one? Why have weeds in your body's garden when you wouldn't have them in your backyard garden? Why have different attitudes about the material things in your life than you do about *your* body, *your* environment?

You may live in many homes, live in many areas of the country, drive many different cars, and you'll certainly wear a lot of different clothes during your lifetime. But you'll live your life inside of just one body. Conduct a spring cleaning. Eliminate all the nasty accumulations of the winter of your life and let in the clean, fresh spring air. Live your life well by constantly rejuvenating it. Mother Nature does it for us in the cycles of the seasons. We are treated to a regeneration of life every year. Treat your body the same way. You'll be energized, rejuvenated, and look and feel better. And everyone around you will look better too. You'll have a more positive outlook and see all those around you in a new light. You'll feel as if everyone else has changed, and yet all the change will have come from within you. Youth is active; it is full of motion created by determination and will. The absence of youth is passivity and resignation. That's why cleaning house and getting rid of all the old notions is such a potent and self-fulfilling activity—you are literally willing yourself younger!

A G E
ERASER

MEET THE MAN IN THE GLASS

Some time ago I read a wonderful little poem that has been part of my life for many years. I have shared it with many friends and asked them to keep it in mind as they pursued their daily activities. Earlier in this chapter I made reference to it and promised you that I would tell you about this poem when I wanted you to understand that the person that you had to take care of was the person you were looking at in the mirror. I first learned of the poem in a story I read about the great baseball pitcher, Herb Score. It's said he has carried a copy of this poem with him since his sophomore year in high school—more than half a century ago.

In the early 1950s, Herb Score was a young phenom pitcher in the Cleveland Indians organization. He was said to throw the baseball faster—in excess of 100 mph—than any pitcher who had come before him. Some experts say he was the Nolan Ryan of his time, with the potential to be one of the greatest pitchers of all time and a sure bet for the Baseball Hall of Fame. Most baseball aficionados expected that Herb Score's legacy would be winning more than 300 games, throwing thousands of strikes, and pitching several no-hitters on his way to a plaque in Cooperstown. That was the expectation of the public—now here's the reality.

On a hot summer night, one of Herb Score's 100-mph fastballs, thrown to New York Yankees shortstop Gil McDougal, came roaring back at him at more than 120 mph. Score was unable to react fast enough to protect himself. The ball hit Score's eye and landed over 200 feet away. Seeing this, most thought this was the end of Herb Score's career. There would be no Hall of Fame, just a footnote in the pages of baseball history. Experiencing this, most people would probably have left the game of baseball and gotten as far away from it as possible. Who would want to be around the game with its tragic memories and reminders of what might have been?

Herb Score was not like most people. He had a different expectation of himself. He believed he could do more than just fill the record books with wins and strikeouts. He believed he knew and loved the game of baseball inside and out, and wanted to help thousands of others to know and love the game as he did. So that night Herb Score picked himself up, and even though he could not play the game he loved, he became the radio voice of the Cleveland Indians for the next 40 years, providing insights and information and bringing the game alive to all of us who sat next to our radios on hot summer nights.

Expectation was that Herb Score would reach the Baseball Hall of Fame in Cooperstown. Reality is that he may well reach the Broadcast Hall of Fame—all because he believed it was not the dreams of others that he had to fulfill. His obligation was to those dreams inside himself. From this rough spot on the pathway of life, Herb Score discovered who he was and what he could do best. When he looked at the man in the glass, and talked to the man in the glass, the man answered back. The rest is history.

Herb Score has told his story to millions of people over the airways and to hundreds of thousands at luncheons, dinners, and banquets; and he always delivers a very positive message. People fortunate enough to hear him speak always say they leave the room inspired, taken by the grace and positive slant he placed on his own misfortune. He was never a bitter man. He was never one who said, "Look what life did to me." He was a man who recognized that he was in control of his own destiny. He knew he had to first satisfy himself. Most people thought his God-given ability was to throw a baseball. Herb Score discovered his ability to share the game he loved and thus he was true to himself and to the poem that he carried with him for years, "The Man in the Glass."

The Guy in the Glass

When you get what you want, in your struggle for pelf
and the world makes you King for a day,
then go to a mirror and look at yourself
and see what that guy has to say.

For it isn't your Father, or Mother, or Wife
who judgment upon you must pass.
The feller whose verdict counts most in your life
is the guy staring back from the glass.

He's the feller to please, never mind all the rest,
for he's with you clear to the end,
and you've passed your most dangerous, difficult test
if the guy in the glass is your friend.

You may be like Jack Horner and "chisel" a plum
and think you're a wonderful guy,
But the man in the glass says you're only a bum
if you can't look him straight in the eye.

You may fool the whole world down the pathway of years
and get pats on your back as you pass,
but your final reward will be heartache and tears
if you've cheated the guy in the glass.

I thank the author of this poem, Dale Wimbrow, because of the contribution he has made to my life and to thousands of others, and if you've not read it before, maybe it will make a contribution to your life.

As you build your relationships and you bring people into your life, remember that you are going to see them as you see the person in this poem. You are going to judge others, love others, treat others, and have an impact on others as you judge the man or woman in the glass. You will be as kind and merciful and as giving in your judgment of others as you will be to the one looking back in the glass.

This is the beginning of a cycle of love and respect that breeds an enduring sense of joy and youthfulness in your life. Anger, jealousy, pettiness, and low self-esteem will turn you into a bitter and feeble old man or woman faster than anything on this earth. When you respect yourself, you start a wonderful and positive cycle that comes back to you throughout your life.

When you feel good about the person you see in the glass, your behavior will reflect that feeling. You won't feed your body junk. You will feed it what it needs, not what the advertiser on television tells you tastes good. You won't accept what the tobacco manufacturer tells you is going to calm your nerves when, in fact, it is going to do just the opposite. You won't feed your body excessive alcohol to deaden your nervous system. You won't abuse it with excessive amounts of fat, or neglect it with inactivity. You won't create or tolerate relationships that bring hostility and negativity into your life. You will understand that it is easier to love than it is to hate, and that it is easier to be kind than it is to be cruel. When your life is filled with positive feelings about yourself and loving relationships with others, your "will to live" and your desire to savor the thrill of life will burn more intensely.

You will make a fundamental decision about how long you are going to live. This decision will be both conscious and unconscious. Your body will get the message. It is no coincidence that people under stress and people whose lives lack positive congruity are more susceptible to disease and early death. How many people do you know whom you almost expect to fall ill, and who then do exactly that?

You can decide to live 140 years, as I have decided to live. Or you can decide, at age 65, that because someone says it's time to retire, you are going to lie down and die. Some people let themselves die inside and refuse to lie down, but either way they are dead. My tone is harsher than usual now, because when I see people who follow this course, I am extremely disappointed. It saddens me that people give up such a wonderfully rich part of their lives and cheat their families out of years of love and happiness.

Not long ago I saw the movie *Pay It Forward*. It is a movie with a simple theme. A young boy put forth the theory that when something nice is done for you, you don't wait to pay *back* the favor. Instead, you pay it *forward*, by doing a good deed for someone else. If something nice is done for you, you aren't to wait for the opportunity to repay the giver—that's not what the person wanted when they did the kind act anyway. You are to pay the favor forward and help out someone else, thus starting a chain reaction of sorts, a chain-letter type of reaction. And with each good act, you will feel better about yourself, your life, and your relationships with others.

As my children grew and began to take control of their lives, they would one by one all ask me what they could do to repay me for the things I'd done as a parent. My answer was simple, "You can't, but you can try to be an even better parent to your children than I was to you." I also tell them I hope that their children will make them as proud as I am of each one of them.

FIND PEACE AND NEVER QUIT

All things are possible if you feel good about yourself and are truly at peace. This will bring harmony to your universe. Throughout this book I've shown you how to bring your body into harmonious balance through many different physical and nutritional activities, allowing you to function at maximum proficiency. If we can bring that same harmonious balance to our mind, then our mental and physical activities, working together, will create so much positive energy in our lives that we cannot help but remain Forever Young!

One of the great examples I can give of the combination of the never-say-die and never-quit attitude regarding you and your relationships and how they affect your success, your beliefs about success, your desire to achieve, and the place of your spiritual beliefs, could not have been better demonstrated than in the 2001 Daytona 500 NASCAR race.

Michael Waltrip comes from a family with a great winning tradition. In this particular race, Michael drove a car owned by Dale Earnhardt, who along with his son, Dale Earnhardt, Jr., was also in the race. All three were members of the Earnhardt team. The statistic that everyone kept repeating during the race was that Michael Waltrip had climbed into his car 462 times to race, and 462 times he ended the race having failed to win. He'd never, ever taken a victory lap in 462 races! His brother Darryl was a winner and champion. On this day, Michael drove on a team of NASCAR legends and winners. And here Michael was starting his 463rd race without a win.

The race was going along just fine, and after 175 clean laps with only a couple of cautions, suddenly 18 or 19 of the cars were involved in an accident. Michael escaped being caught in any of the collisions, and after a red flag temporarily stopped the race, he quickly worked himself into the lead, with Dale Earnhardt, Jr., right behind him, and Dale Earnhardt, Sr., following both of them, fending off challengers so that his two teammates could stay in front. Earnhardt, Sr., the man known as a fierce competitor and nicknamed "the intimidator," had made a decision. He was using his superior racing skills to block the rest of the driving field from getting around him to take victory from Dale, Jr., and

Michael Waltrip. Earnhardt, Sr., was actually going to assist and allow his teammates to win, a move totally outside of his normal racing character. A more human, and certainly less selfish, spirit had taken over at that moment.

On the next to the last lap, Dale Earnhardt, Sr., was involved in a collision that appeared not to be as severe as many he'd walked away from, and Michael Waltrip crossed the finish line with his first win in 463 attempts. And it was not only his first NASCAR win, it was the prestigious Daytona 500, long recognized as one of the premier NASCAR races.

You don't have to be a racing fan to appreciate this story. It's a great life success story. It's the story of a man who never quit. And at the end of the race he put all of the issues I've written about here right out front. He was spiritual. He said he wanted to thank God. And then he turned around and said he wanted to love and hug the Earnhardts for having faith in him, for making him a part of their lives and their team. And he wanted to thank his father, the man he wished could be there, because this was such an important event and he wanted to share it with him. Michael's brother, acting as a commentator for Fox TV, had tears in his eyes as he watched his brother finally win. All the elements I've talked about were there: the interaction of relationships, spiritual guidance, and an unfailing belief in oneself.

And tragically, the perfect example of living life to its fullest, right down to the last moment of your life was there too. The crash that didn't appear to be as bad as some others, took the life of Dale Earnhardt, Sr. He was killed instantly as he hit the wall, racing as hard as he always did and protecting the lead of his teammates. He died living his life exactly as he wanted to. Everyone who knew and loved him knows that to be the truth. That was their solace during their time of grief.

I believe that you and I are God's greatest miracles. I repeat this in nearly every episode of my television show. Why is this so important to me? Because you have to respect such a magnificent gift. This is reflected in the way you treat others, and in the way you treat yourself. Your body is a temple. It is where you can accomplish what you want.

Again, I'm not writing a book about religion and am not recruiting you to subscribe to a particular faith, or believe as I do. I just want to encourage you to recognize the need for a spiritual side to your life. I always stress that in order to remain Forever Young, you have to be young in mind, young in body, and young in spirit. You do not have to share my religious beliefs or any religious beliefs at all. You simply have to believe that inside of you there exists the ability to be the best that you can possibly be. Because it is in turning your goals into the visions you see of yourself that you will become your best self. You must constantly stimulate your brain, maintain your body, and nourish the spiritual side of your life in order to be the well-rounded and harmonious being you want to be.

MAKE A PROMISE TO YOURSELF

I believe that you can be the fountain of youth. I believe you are the perfect miracle. All that you have to do is make a promise to yourself. Don't promise me. This is not about me. So begin right here. Write your name in the blank space below right now.

> I, _____, [Don't read on until you sign your name here. Did you write it down?] accept my inalienable right, given to me by a higher power, to take control of my total destiny, to see light where there is darkness, to bring joy where there is sadness, to instill love where it is not understood, to show kindness when it is lacking, to understand when understanding is needed, to bring patience to tasks where anything less would be futile, and to be true to the gifts that have been given to me by my creator.
>
> I make this promise to myself, at this very moment, to take control and instill the following into my life: I promise to put love above all other things, to put loyalty right behind it, to be committed to excellence—not to be better than others or to win—but to discover who and what I am and then commit myself to be the best that I can be, and to take these wonderful gifts and use them for the good of all.

BEGIN A PROGRAM FOR LIFE

If you can make this promise to yourself, if you can follow this vow, you will wake up tomorrow morning with renewed vigor, boundless energy, and you will be on the path to remaining Forever Young. *You will decide to start a program for life.* You will begin to make proper nutrition part of your everyday diet plan. You will *make* the time to exercise and you will find that it will give you more time to spend with your loved ones and to be more effective on your job. You will make time to help others and to bring joy to all around you.

You will soon discover that this approach to life can melt wrinkles in your brow as fast as the methods I discussed in the skin-care chapter. You will have the dynamic energy to go out and exercise, whether it's lifting weights, playing tennis, running track, or swimming laps.

You will bring living into the word *life*. You won't just be existing. You will wake up every day with a zest for living, grateful for the opportunity to give again. You will ask yourself, "What can I do today to remain Forever Young?" You will go through every day knowing that you are now doing the most joyful thing on this planet—giving all you have to give and experiencing every moment. You will live every moment and not just exist. You're not just passing through this life; you are making an impact. It's *your* world, and your world will turn out the way you want it to *because you are taking control.*

You see, Forever Young is more than a phrase. I can't leave you at the end of this book thinking that it is some kind of narcissistic statement from someone who thinks that they just have to be pretty, handsome, and youthful—that is not what Forever Young is about. It's about the exuberance and the acceptance and the joy that you knew as a child. It's that innocence, that love you gave freely to everyone before others began to spoil it. It is that voice within you that said you could do anything, you could try anything.

Remember those days? "You're young," people would say, dismissing your unbridled innocence and enthusiasm for life. How often do you hear the phrase, "You know when I was young I would . . ." Well, isn't your life still flush with opportunities? Don't you still have the ability to dream and the vitality to reach for those dreams? Don't answer that too quickly unless your answer is a simple *yes*. Otherwise, you are going to answer it incorrectly. I know that you still have the ability to recapture your youthful vitality. I have shown you some ways in this book; some through modern science and some through more natural ways. I have told you about methods science can document and prove, and some anecdotal techniques that you can only prove by trying them yourself and finding out how they work for you.

I will remain a conduit to this information, bringing it to you through my television show, our age-management seminars, our tapes, our clinics, our newsletters, our products, and our web site, **BillFrank'sForeverYoung.com.** Whatever, whenever, and in every way that I can, I will share with you the many ways to stay Forever Young.

When it comes to turning your life around, I want you to recapture that fearless, almost reckless attitude of your youth. Do you remember what it was like when you weren't afraid to try something new? Do you remember when you were not afraid to try? You thought, "What the heck. I might as well try. No one's going to shoot me if I don't make it. It's not life or death."

As a child we get knocked down and we get right back up and keep on trying. That's one of the wonders of youth. We aren't concerned with failure. But as we get older we seem to become more timid about trying anything that might not turn out the way we want it to. You'll never know how anything will turn out if you don't give it a chance. It's hard to be a participant in life when you're sitting in the grandstands watching all the action. Experience is the only way to learn about and change your life—the only way to learn how to take care of yourself.

TAKE CARE OF YOUR MIND, BODY, AND SPIRIT

For your part, I am asking you in some ways to become a *selfish* person. This doesn't mean to neglect others—actually it's the opposite. I want you to take care of *you* first. If you take care of yourself, then you can begin to take care of the people around you. A man sitting in the street without two nickels to rub together has nothing to contribute to charity. He can't help build any foundations. He can't give shelter to the homeless—he is the homeless and he needs help. This man does, however, create the opportunity for the person who has accomplished much in his life to step forward and help someone less fortunate.

I'm sure you're familiar with the safety announcement made at the beginning of all airline flights. It says that if an unexpected change in cabin pressure occurs, oxygen masks will drop from a panel in the overhead compartment. You are instructed to first put on and adjust *your* oxygen mask before helping those around you, even if you are traveling with an infant. *You can be of no assistance to anyone if you don't first take care of yourself.*

If you have received much from life, I believe you are obligated to give some of it back. If you have learned how to take care of your mind, your body, and your spirit, I believe you should want to reach out and help those who haven't yet learned how to do that. I believe this is when you should *pay it forward.* And you will be able to do just that as a result of being *selfish*—taking care of yourself first so that you are then *able* to help others.

If your life is limited owing to preventable illness, or if you leave this world prematurely, you are depriving others of the joy you might bring to their lives. I recently attended the funeral of a 58-year-old woman who was taken from her loved ones in the prime of her life and vitality. Somehow, unknown to her, her immune system had withered, and a very manageable disease took her life. I experienced the profound sadness of her husband and children, whose plans and dreams were cut so many years short.

Someone who is sick and depressed will not be able to help or heal anyone else. They are simply not able to lift anyone's spirit. But those with a healthy body, mind, and spirit—and the desire to share—can make a magnificent difference in people's lives.

In 1972 I was running a health spa in Garden Grove, California. One day, an extremely obese 43-year-old woman came into my office. Now I wish that I had the money to build health clubs all over the world and let everyone come in and use them for free. But I don't, and that's not the way the world works. So I talked with the woman about the cost of a membership in the spa, she told to me that she just couldn't afford the $17 monthly fee it would cost her to join. She explained that she had three children that she had to care for and eventually put through college. I tried to tell her that she needed to take care of herself first and in doing so be better able to take care of her children.

At that time I was a few years younger than the woman, but I still realized that she was young and had a lot of living ahead of her. I wanted her to lose weight and get healthy—in short, to take care of herself. I did my best. I'm sure there are even those who would say that I used some high-pressure sales tactics. My tactics must have made some impression, because she went home and told her sons what I had said to her. I even talked to her two more times on the phone. I asked her what would happen if, because of her poor physical condition, she wasn't around long enough to care for her family. However, my words didn't seem to have an impact on her, and she didn't join the health club.

Less than a year later, a young man I did not know and whose name I did not recognize, came into the health club and asked to see me. To be honest, I was busy, and tried to put him off, but he persisted. He said he wanted to tell me a story that he "thought would make me work harder," and would certainly make him feel better. I wasn't sure if I should be offended, but he had piqued my curiosity so I invited him to sit down.

He told me the story of a 43-year-old extremely obese woman who had come to my health club the year before, who had even cried in my office and later at home because she thought I was being mean to her. I remembered her because she was so grossly obese, and because she had won the battle that day. Her tears had made me feel bad enough that I quit trying to convince her that she needed to take care of herself.

As fate would have it, she won the battle with me, but lost the war with life. Her son told me that she had died from a heart attack in her sleep and that he and his brothers had found her the next morning. I asked him why he wanted to tell me this story. He said it was because she had come home from seeing me, crying and telling him all of the terrible things I had said to her. He told me that I had hurt her feelings. Of course I felt bad. I told him I was sorry about his mother and sorry if I had hurt her, but I could not remember what specifically I had said to her. He said, "You told her the truth, Mr. Frank. You told her that while she thought she was doing everything for us boys, she really wasn't. You asked her what would happen to us if she was gone. You told her that if she didn't do something about her weight she wouldn't be around to see us graduate from college. And more than that, you asked her who would be there to pay for our schooling and take care of us."

Well, all of that happened, and the young man told me he had just been forced to leave his freshman year of college and come home to help care for his younger brothers. He told me he loved his mother, but also realized that if she'd cut the grocery bill by $17 each month, and spent it on a spa membership for herself, and if she'd come into the spa every week and taken off some weight, increased her circulation, and eased her breathing—she still might be there with her sons.

The young man told me he wanted to study physical therapy. He wanted people to understand that one of the best things they can do for those they love is to take care of themselves first. He said he didn't want other children to have to bury a young mother. And he said again that he wanted me to work harder the next time someone like his mother came into my health club. That young man brought tears to my eyes. He made me feel terrible about letting his mother leave without a health-club membership. I had let her walk out that day knowing that she was cutting her life short. *I hadn't worked hard enough.*

I currently work in a world where I am frequently given the opportunity to help people improve their health, and you better believe I don't quit until I know I've done my best to help them start turning their life around! That young man's story made a big impact on my life. I learned by graphic example that we must help ourselves before we can help anyone else. I hope you don't have a lot of stories like this one in your life. They are so sad. But if you do have some event like that in your past, then learn from it and promise yourself to do better at the next opportunity.

UNDERSTAND THE REAL MEANING OF FOREVER YOUNG

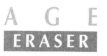

I'm trying to make a difference. If this book reaches out and touches the lives of just a few people who will go out and touch the lives of a few more—soon thousands of people will understand that Forever Young is not just somebody's narcissistic idea of existing forever.

I don't believe that people who wake up depressed and dispirited can muster the motivation to steadfastly choose the right foods and engage in a healthy lifestyle during the course of that day. In fact, when I meet a person who is overweight, exhausted from overwork, out of breath from walking up a few stairs, hunched over without even the strength of will to stand erect, I ask myself, "What is their spiritual crisis? Why are they unhappy? Why do they view themselves as so unworthy?"

I believe the answer lies in the word that describes their state—*dis*pirited, or *without* spirit. If you don't feel your relationship with your creator or personal higher power is providing a greater spiritual value to your life, you may never feel the real joy of life or understand the real meaning of being Forever Young. If you can't answer that you are doing all that you can for others, or that you are doing all that you can do to actualize your own potential, you will neglect your most vital needs.

That's why, in closing, I want to remind you again of the words, "Love thy neighbor as thyself." If that's the standard I'm trying to live by, then what am I doing if I don't begin by loving the man in the glass? If the man or woman looking back at you is not someone you love, then you are going to take it out on yourself mentally and physically. You won't eat right. You won't exercise. You won't get enough rest. You won't be energized. You won't have much to give to others. And you certainly won't be able to remain Forever Young.

Never once in this book did I tell you that you would exist forever. All that we have talked about is that whatever *your* forever is—however many years you are in this miracle of a body that God has given you—you must respect it. You are not just renting space. You are not simply leasing it. You cannot give back a broken-down, wretched mess and pick out a new one from the showroom. If you owned a home and you let it run down, what would it be worth? Well, this home that you are living in—the one that you call your body—that's the one that you have to maintain. The longer you take care of it, the longer you can live there. You will live in many brick-and-mortar homes, but you are only going to live in one body. Take care of your body. Take care of your mind, and all the wonderful intricate systems in your body. And most importantly, take care of your spiritual side.

AGE ERASER

STEP OUT OF THE OLD AND INTO THE NEW

You've probably heard a lot of books in the self-help genre talk about "60 days to turn your life around," or "10 weeks to lose 10 pounds," or "30 days to greatness." I'm here to tell you that you can make a fundamental change in your life in 19 seconds! Did you sign your name on the line a few pages ago? How long did it take you to make that decision, to make that vow? That's how long it took you to step out of the old and into the new. That's how long it took you to change your life.

It means that you won't read this book and say, "Oh, this is a good book—good for somebody else." No. You understand that this book is *personally for you.* The message is directed to the person who signed on the line—you. You don't have to do all of the things that we tell you about. Simply use this book to help you decide what is best for you. Let it lead you to other research. Let it lead you to the point in your life where you make the commitment to be Forever Young—to not accept tired old ideas or somebody telling you at what point in time you have to shut down, or what you can or can't do. *You* be the one to decide. *You* make the decisions. *You* take the lead.

Since most of the things that I have done in my life have been based on faith—I am asking you to have a little bit of faith too. Not in me, but in yourself, and in the principles that have filled these pages. Antiaging science today is remarkable. The techniques are available for you. The proof has been provided again and again. You can slow down the clock. You can even reverse the clock. You can squeeze so much more joy from life, once you toss away your preconceptions of the inevitability of aging.

Anyone who's lost a loved one too early, or tragically seen lives destroyed by illness, will understand my motivation for writing this book. I've experienced a lot in my nearly six decades of living, some good and some bad. But I do know this today: my unspoken prayers have been answered. I have been richly blessed with knowledge and, as a result, I have written a book—not as someone who knows more than you, but as an individual who has compiled a wealth of information about holding onto life, and who knows that it is now time to share it, as so many others have been so kind and generous over the years to share with me. As I previously mentioned, I have known some great scientists, celebrities, athletes, individuals from all walks of life who have shared their stories and their secrets with me, and I have shared this information here with you.

You may do with this information what you wish. But if you take away nothing else from this book, please remember this: love yourself, control your destiny, be willing to believe that you are God's greatest miracle, and most of all, that you are intended to remain Forever Young.

Representation by
    Daniel J. Levin
    Levin Entertainment Co.
    532 Colorado Avenue
    Santa Monica, CA 90401
    310-576-7000
    310-576-4900

Exercise Photographs
    Dale Bush
    bushd@metatec.com

REFERENCES AND RESOURCES

American Academy of Facial Plastic and Reconstructive Surgery
310 S. Henry St.
Alexandria, VA 22314
800-332-FACE
www.facial-plastic-surgery.org
e-mail: info@aafprs.org

American Board of Facial Plastic and Reconstructive Surgery
115C S. Saint Asaph St.
Alexandria, VA 22314
703-549-3223
www.abfprs.org

American Sleep Disorders Association
1610 14th St. NW
Suite 300
Rochester, MN 55901
507-287-6006
www.asda.org

Jean Berry
LifeCell Technologies, Inc.
3172 Virginia St.

Coconut Grove, FL 33133
305-774-0340
www.lifecell.net

Cenegenics Medical Institute
851 S. Rampart Blvd.
Las Vegas, NV 89128
Dr. Alan Mintz, Founder
Dr. David Leonardi, Medical Director
888-YOUNGER
www.888younger.com

Bill Frank and Forever Young Products, Club, Information
www.billfranksforeveryoung.com

Firm Fitness
Sam and Angela Velez
Pompano Beach, FL
954-784-4646

Healthfinder
www.healthfinder.gov
A government-sponsored gateway site for online information sponsored by
the U.S. Department of Health and Human Services. Provides links to
federal, state, and local agencies, not-for-profit organizations, and
universities.

National Institutes of Health
9000 Rockville Pike
Bethesda, MD 20892
301-496-1776
www.nih.gov

National Mental Health Association
1021 Prince St.
Alexandria, VA 22314
800-969-NMHA
www.nmha.org

National Osteoporosis Foundation
1150 17th St. NW
Suite 500

Washington, DC 20036
800-223-9994
www.nof.org

Bill Pearl Enterprises, Inc.
PO Box 1080
Phoenix, OR 97535
541-535-3363
www.billpearl.com

Dr. Jim Shortt
Age and Sports Medicine Specialist
W. Columbia, SC
803-755-0114

Brad Sorenson
Healthcare Marketing Services
Ft. Lauderdale, FL
800-390-6134

Beryl Wolk
Beryl's World
Jenkinstown, PA
www.berylsworld.com

World Gym
Jim Lorimer and Gary Benford
Columbus, OH
614-430-5962

Dr. David Zipfel
10506 Montgomery Road
Suite 101
Cincinnati, OH 45242
513-793-1171

index

niacin (Vitamin B$_3$), skin care and, 87

nitrogen, 32
  energy and, 138
nootropics, 7, 117, 119–121
Norman, Greg, 2
  nutrition value of common foods, 47–48. *See also* diet

Octoplasty, 92
Omega-3 essential fatty acids, 139–140
orange juice, 125–127
organotherapy. *See* live cell therapy
osteoblasts, 181
osteoclasts, 181
osteoporosis, 96
  folic acid and, 109
  live cell therapy and, 197–198
  progesterone and, 181–182
oxidation, 115, 122

PABA, 86
Parker, Dave, 52, 137
Parkinson's disease, 115
Parrish, Lance, 52
Passwater, Richard, 132
pau d'arco, 17–18
Pay It Forward, 219
Pearl, Bill, 57
phenol peel, 92
phosphatidylserine, 120
phosphorus, 110
physicians, antiaging, 186–187
phytochemicals, 127–128
phytoestrogens, 160
Piracetam, 121
plastic surgery, 91–93
polycythemia, 175–176
potassium, 127–128

power peels, 92
pregnenolone, 120, 155–156
Premarin, 178
progesterone, 181–182
Propecia, 177
Proscar, 177
prostate health, 160–161, 176–177
  DHT and, 176–177
  testosterone and, 173
protein
  energy conversion and, 137–138
  muscle nourishment and, 54
  60–percent solution and, 30–31
protein/nitrogen balance, 138
pumpkin seed oil, 161
push-pull exercise theory, 58–61
pycnogenol, 131–132
pygeum, 160
pyroglutamic acid, brain health and, 119

Reading, brain health and, 118
Reinsdorf, Jerry, 79
Reiter, R. J., 184
relationships, 202–229
  environmental control and, 213
  knowledge of self and, 214–216
  life program and, 222–224
  peace and, 220–222
respiratory infections, 128
Restak, Richard, 113
Retinol/Retin A, 89, 128
rhinoplasty, 92
rhytidectomy, 92
Riggs, B. L., 181
Ryan, Nolan, 52, 137

Williams, Venus, 53
Wimbrow, Dale, 218
Wolkowitz DHEA study, 171
women
    calcium and, 108
    cancer and, 27
    estrogen decline and, 147
    exercise and, 51
    heart disease prevention and, 126
    menopause and, 146, 171, 182

testosterone and, 172
weight training and, 52, 54
Wyeth-Ayerst, 179

Yohimbine, 156–157

Zinc, 109, 160